AF831165

CHAZZ **WEAVER**, Ph.D-C
50, FIT, & FABULOUS

THE O.C. DIET REVOLUTION

REVEALING THE MYSTERY OF WEIGHT LOSS

FOREWORD BY **RUTH KAVA,** Ph.D., R.D.
DIRECTOR OF NUTRITION,
AMERICAN COUNCIL ON SCIENCE AND HEALTH

The OC Diet Revolution

Revealing the mystery of weight loss

Chazz Weaver Ph.D-C

50, Fit & Fabulous

Tate Publishing & *Enterprises*

TATE PUBLISHING
& Enterprises

The OC Diet Revolution

Copyright © 2006 by Chazz Weaver, Ph.D-C. All rights reserved.

No part of this publication may be reproduced, stored in a retrieval system or transmitted in any way by any means, electronic, mechanical, photocopy, recording or otherwise without the prior permission of the author except as provided by USA copyright law.

The opinions expressed by the author are not necessarily those of Tate Publishing, LLC.

This book is designed to provide accurate and authoritative information with regard to the subject matter covered. This information is given with the understanding that neither the author nor Tate Publishing, LLC is engaged in rendering legal, professional advice. Since the details of your situation are fact dependent, you should additionally seek the services of a competent professional.

Book design copyright © 2006 by Tate Publishing, LLC. All rights reserved.

Cover design by Leah LeFlore
Layout design by Rusty Eldred
Cover photo by: Michael Neveux

Published in the United States of America

ISBN: 1-5988695-4-X

06.10.31

TABLE OF CONTENTS

FOREWORD

As a professional nutritionist, I sometimes despair when reading about popular weight loss diets. Every other week, it seems, there is a new diet book with a new gimmick that promises fast weight loss with no effort. No calorie counting, no exercise, no sweat! But the truth is, of course, that calories do count, physical activity is important, and a healthy lifestyle does not just happen without some thought and preparation. At last, though, someone is telling it like it is. Chazz Weaver, economist and fitness coach, got tired of the hype and misinformation typically dished out in the guise of nutrition and health advice and decided to present the truth.

I became acquainted with Chazz when he embarked on his 30-day McDonald's diet challenge, in response to the media hyperbole about the supposed deadly nature of fast-foods. I evaluated the nutritional composition of the diet he consumed, based on his careful records of every bite. I found, as I had expected, that he was able to derive pretty much all his necessary nutrients from his McDonald's sojourn, and improve some important health markers as well.

In *The OC Diet Revolution* Chazz gives the reader the tools with which to figure out his or her individual diet and exercise plan. More than that, though, he explains why our modern environment and lifestyle make it so difficult for many to reach and maintain a healthy weight—how our metabolism evolved to deal with a very different set of challenges.

Unlike other diet book authors, Chazz doesn't stop with explaining the whys and hows of weight loss and fitness. He acknowledges the significant impact of social and psychological factors on food choices and consumption, and encourages the reader to take these into account. Chazz doesn't try to impose any one system on readers, rather, he encourages individuals to find a motivational plan that will work for them—one that takes into account their own preferences and lifestyles.

As an entrepreneur, family man, and fitness practitioner, Chazz Weaver does not just talk the talk—he's not another paunchy weight control guru who says, "Do as I say, not as I do." Indeed, the man walks the walk, and will help others join him on the path to health.

The OC Diet Revolution is not a book to read once and consign to the shelf; it's a reference book on healthful living—one that readers will want to keep checking again and again for all the valuable tips and insights it offers.

Ruth Kava, Ph.D., R.D.
Director of Nutrition,
American Council on Science and Health
New York, NY

A FUNDAMENTAL TRUTH

The OC Diet Revolution is the bedrock from which all weight loss programs are derived; its foundation is a mathematical truth:

Calories + Anaerobic Activities + Aerobic Activities = Body Composition

Your body, healthy or not, is a direct result of these components. The decision to over-eat and not exercise involves a trade-off between short-term benefits of consumption and the long-term costs to future health. Therefore, while the effects of obesity are a burden on the health care system, the factors associated with obesity are an economic issue.

Chazz Weaver Ph.D-C

WHY YOU NEED TO READ THIS BOOK

Are You a Casualty of the Diet Industry's Empty Promises?

If you are reading this, you may be one of the 190 million Americans who are overweight or obese. If you are not overweight, the information contained in the confines of this text can elevate you to a new level of fitness. However, if you are like most other adults facing the challenge of being overweight or obese, you have probably looked to a number of sources trying to select the best approach to solve your problem. Even though success has eluded you up to this point, you are to be applauded for your efforts. By taking the initiative and researching diets and fitness programs, you have shown that you are ready to make a change in your life. Good for you! Unfortunately, the quality of fitness and health information that has been available to most consumers in recent years has been insufficient.

The diet industry in the United States is a vast, highly profitable sector of the economy. It is estimated to be responsible for over fifty billion dollars in annual revenue. Men and women struggling with their weight are faced with a mind-boggling array of programs and regimens.

If you are standing in the diet section of the bookstore as you are reading this book, a quick glance up and down the aisle will reveal the scope of the diet regimens, programs, and fads that have captured the

American imagination in recent years: The Zone Diet, the Atkins Diet, the South Beach Diet, Body for Life, Sugar Busters, and Dr. Phil's Weight Loss Solution are just a few of the most prominent contenders that constitute the tip of a very large iceberg.

We have been bombarded with tales of how people in France, Greece, Italy, and other countries and cultures feast on their native cuisines without succumbing to the obesity epidemic that is facing the United States. We have gone from being told that low-fat diets were the only approach to lasting weight loss to being informed that, in truth, it was the carbohydrates in our food that were responsible for our ever-expanding waistlines. Now, the low-carbohydrate backlash has begun, and the conventional wisdom of weight-loss appears to be swinging back towards the low-fat approach.

The back-and-forth advice of the weight-loss industry can make even the most nutritionally-informed consumer feel like a spectator in the audience at Wimbledon. It's enough to make your head spin! Ironically, even as the rate and prevalence of overweight and obesity in the United States has continued to skyrocket, the number of weight loss programs and so-called experts persist to increase exponentially, as well. For a society that is growing more overweight by the year, we seem to have an insatiable appetite for new weight loss programs!

Believe me, I am not making light of the real struggles and challenges facing men and women with weight problems. Instead, what I *am* fed up with is the misleading, confusing, and sometimes outright *false* information that has been served to the American public by the increasingly profitable diet industry. If you think about it, the diet industry only serves to ensure its own survival and continued success by confusing consumers. If I were a more cynical person, I might even begin to believe that the diet industry conspires to perpetuate confusion among American consumers in order to make sure that their books, programs, guides, supplements, meal bars and shakes, calendars, cookbooks, and hundreds of other products continue to sell.

The truth of the matter is much less exciting. Instead, much of the information peddled by the diet industry is simply the modern-day equivalent of the snake-oil salesmen and tonic peddlers that used to take advantage of people back in the old days. Obesity is the greatest health threat facing the United States today, to mention nothing of the emotional and social problems that being overweight causes for millions of men, women, and children. Like a greedy, bloated vampire, the diet industry continues to feed on the desperate struggle that overweight individuals often experience.

Another Harmful Diet Industry Strategy: Calling Personal Responsibility into Question

During the same period that obesity reached epidemic proportions in the United States, a troubling trend began to emerge in which social conditions began to take the primary blame for our collective weight problem. The first widely recognizable sign of this trend was the wave of lawsuits filed against food manufacturers and fast-food companies in the 1990s. Though the facts of each case differed, the gist of these lawsuits was that people had been duped by these companies into overeating, leading to a lifetime of obesity, health problems, and diminished quality of life.

I am not going to name all of the logical inconsistencies in this argument; nor am I going to lecture you at length about my personal ideology. However, I have a real problem with the notion that we should so easily give up our sense of personal responsibility for our weight problems, choosing instead to place the blame on familiar societal and corporate scapegoats.

This is not to say that eating fast-food, or any food for that matter, consistently and in large quantities will not make you fat; on the contrary, I think that any rational adult probably recognizes that as a fact. What does bother me about laying the blame for obesity on food companies and other corporate entities is that it removes any degree of personal investment in one's own health. And when you willingly give up a sense of personal responsibility for your own health and fitness, you may also start to believe that you have no control over these variables.

What I want to tell you—and what I will tell you in this book—is that you *do* have control over your weight, fitness, health, and quality of life. I want to give you the tools and knowledge that you need to take control of these things, regain your health, and maximize your happiness and enjoyment of life. I feel so strongly about the importance of these tools that I have founded a not-for-profit organization **www.truthinfitness.org** that is wholly dedicated to spreading the truth about diet, health, and fitness.

Although individuals have been primarily responsible for the lawsuits that have been filed against fast-food companies and other food providers charging them with contributing to the obesity epidemic, I feel that the diet industry has also further extended the harmful perspective that minimizes personal responsibility for weight gain. The diet industry has done this in two ways: first, by using emotional appeals that are big on manipulation and exploitation (and short on factual, scientific information) in order to draw in consumers, and secondly, by overemphasizing psychological variables in the weight loss process. The end result has been that many overweight and obese individuals have no idea about the physiological, scientifically established facts that show the factors that contribute to obesity and that must be changed in order to achieve lasting weight loss.

How This Book Will Help You

How is this book different from the other books, products, and gimmicks that have promised to help you regain your health and fitness and then failed to deliver? As a self-taught diet industry "outsider," I consider myself uniquely suited to deserve your trust and lead you through the process of weight loss and increased fitness.

- I adhere strictly to the same type of diet and fitness fundamentals that I am suggesting that you should use. Unlike many of the leading "experts" in the field, I would never ask you to commit to do anything that I myself can't, won't, or don't do.

- Unlike many of the most prominent figures in the diet industry, I am not tainted with any associations, business relationships, or cross-promotion deals within the industry, a situation that often leads to the dissemination of confusing or false fitness information. Instead, I head a non-profit organization that is dedicated to helping men and women like you navigate through the haze of health and fitness confusion and misinformation that is out there.

- Unlike many long-established leaders in the diet industry, my approach to diet, health, and fitness is decidedly down-to-earth and based on my own understanding and experience of real life. I have heard many men and women complain that a number of the recently popular diet plans seem to assume that everyone has a personal chef, unlimited free time, an unrestricted food budget, and a personal gym. I own and manage my own (non-fitness-related) firm, have a family, and I am currently pursuing my PhD. I know first-hand the challenges that real families encounter on a daily basis, and I have developed an approach to diet and fitness that takes these responsibilities into consideration.

- Unlike many popular diet plans, my approach is not based on outlandish, unhealthy nutritional restrictions that would only work in the long-term if you lived alone (with your personal chef, of course) on an uninhabited desert island. Real life means variability in your food intake and options, and this diet takes everyday changes into account. This plan will show you how to make good food choices whether you are cooking dinner for your family at home, dining at a nice restaurant, or making a quick dash through the nearest fast-food drive-thru.

- This book does not contain long lists of exotic, expensive "approved" foods and complicated gourmet recipes. In fact, I am not advocating any specific foods or a certain strictly defined nutritional practice. Instead, I want to provide you with a nutritional decision-making framework that will help you make strong, beneficial food choices anywhere and in any situation.
- The diet and fitness information that will be presented in this book is based on the findings that have been reported in recent scientific data on weight loss and fitness. Unlike other recently popular fad diets that reject the scientific literature and facts as a gimmick that is supposed to reflect the plan's "renegade" status, my approach is firmly rooted in scientific fact and sound, widely accepted medical practices.

What's to Come: An Overview

In contrast to some of the overly complicated diet and fitness plans that crowd the market today, this book will offer a simple, but scientifically sound approach that you can adapt to your own needs, limitations, and circumstances. Only the fundamentals need to remain unchanged; you should feel free to adapt them to your needs. In my experience, the twists and turns of real life require an adaptable approach, and as such, the degree of flexibility in a diet and fitness plan often determines its long-term success.

However, in order to achieve lasting weight loss, increased physical fitness, and an improved quality of life, you must first understand how and why the human body is prone to obesity, as well as how and why so many of the food choices and lifestyles of the twenty-first century tend to promote being overweight or obese. We will explore the eating and exercise habits of our prehistoric ancestors in order to get a better handle on the way that our bodies process food today. In this way, you will be able to manipulate your body's metabolic processes to achieve and maintain permanent weight loss and optimal physical fitness.

When you are done reading this book, you will understand the following principles:

1. The quantity of calories is just as important as the quality;
2. A minimum of aerobic exercise makes weight loss much more efficient;
3. Anaerobic exercise is just as important as aerobic and both have a synergistic effect that will improve the efficiency and effectiveness of any weight loss and weight maintenance program;
4. There is no substitute for the first three principles: no shortcuts, magic elixirs, or instant results.

If you are overweight or out of shape, you have probably sought out other approaches to health and fitness in the past, only to be failed by empty promises, questionable claims, and manipulation. You have been let down, you may have even let *yourself* down, and you are still looking for an answer. I acknowledge and respect that persistence, and I want to help you succeed this time.

As the rate of obesity increases in the United States, the number of products and gimmicks designed to offer the promise of a quick fix seems to increase every day. I want nothing more than to help Americans cut through the misinformation and confusion that is out there. I want to help you design a flexible, realistic, scientifically sound fitness and diet plan that fits the demands of real life.

That's my agenda.

MY JOURNEY THROUGH THE GOLDEN ARCHES

Flip through a recent issue of a general-interest magazine or watch the health and fitness segment of a national newscast, and you will likely run into the kind of black-and-white, all-or-nothing thinking about obesity, diet, exercise, and nutrition that has long been a personal pet peeve of mine. The overly simplistic approach that is often parroted in the mainstream media holds that fitness can only be achieved if one adheres to a strict, often unrealistic eating plan.

The popularity of this point of view reached a fever pitch in the spring of 2004. With a specific focus on fast-food restaurants, the media seemed to be suggesting with increasing regularity that convenience-oriented foods had no place whatsoever in a healthy lifestyle.

Now, it goes without saying that we would all be better served to limit our intake of fast-foods and rely primarily on fresh fruits and vegetables, whole-grain carbohydrates, and lean meat proteins for our daily caloric needs. However, taking into consideration the often-hectic pace of modern life, this type of eating plan is simply unrealistic.

Also, I think that the media's promotion of this point of view encourages too many Americans to take an all-or-nothing approach about their nutrition: if they are too busy to eat healthy foods for every meal, many people tend to throw their hands up in surrender and allow themselves to fall off the deep end of unhealthy eating choices. My own preference is for an approach that promotes healthy foods, but is flexible enough to accommodate some meals from the drive-thru when your schedule becomes extremely busy or unforeseen circumstances demand a quick fix for the occasional lunch or dinner.

Another part of the media's health and fitness information that really bothers me is its tendency to ignore the fundamentals of weight loss. You can make the issue of health and fitness extremely complex by adding in dimensions such as emotions, society, economics, psychology, and culture, or by questioning the value of certain food groups that are high in carbohydrates. At the root, the processes that cause both weight gain and weight loss are extremely basic.

To put it simply, weight gain occurs when you consistently consume more calories than you expend. Conversely, weight loss occurs when you consistently consume fewer calories than you expend. From this perspective, the type of food that you choose to eat does not matter as much in the equation of weight loss as the quantity of food and the amount of exercise that you get each day.

By focusing so extensively on the dangers associated with certain types of food, such as fast-food, I believe that the media has created a great deal of confusion among Americans. The basic equation of weight loss has been lost in the hysteria surrounding which types of food you can and cannot eat. Taking into consideration the epidemic of obesity that this country is dealing with, I feel that spreading this kind of misinformation is dangerous and irresponsible.

To get back to the spring of 2004, the media was engaged in an unusually vigorous denunciation of fast-food. To hear the news reports on the subject, one bite of a Big Mac could cause instant obesity and ill gotten health. Matters were not helped by the publicity machine surrounding the release of a popular, but sensationalistic documentary that depicted what could happen to your body if you ate vast amounts of fast-food for a month while engaging in no exercise or physical exertion whatsoever.

My personal mission has long been focused on improving the health and fitness knowledge and understanding of both myself and the people around me. In the early 2000s, I began to consider ways that I could start working on these goals on a broader scale. This led me to develop a non-profit organization geared towards dispensing objective, factual information about fitness and weight loss to the general public.

All of these factors came together for me in the spring of 2004. Disgusted with the confusion and misinformation about health and fitness that were constantly being conveyed by the mainstream media, I decided to counter some of the hysteria with my own 30-day foray into fast-food eating.

Walking the Walk

The diet that I began on April 1, 2004, included many self-imposed elements and guidelines that will be familiar to people who were following the media hubbub over fast-food in general and McDonald's in particular that year. Some of the rules were different, because my own McDonald's diet was geared toward demonstrating that exercise could offset many of the adverse effects of fast-food meals. For the 30-day period of the diet, I allowed myself to eat only items from the regular McDonald's menu. In addition, I decided that I would eat each menu item at least one time during the month.

Where my plan diverged from other accounts of similar diets was in exercise. I determined that I would stick to my normal daily exercise routine during the 30-day diet. My normal routine consists of 20 minutes of aerobic exercise and 50 minutes of anaerobic exercise (primarily focused on weightlifting).

By the end of the 30-day period, I had lost 8 pounds of body fat and my health had improved in some measures. During the time that I was eating nothing but McDonald's food, I was able to lower my LDL (bad cholesterol) by 2 points and raise my HDL (good cholesterol) by 80%. More importantly, I was successful in my objective of challenging the conventional wisdom that holds fast-food as the primary source of the growing obesity epidemic both in the United States and around the world.

My personal journey through the golden arches of fast-food was motivated by my frustration with the misinformation dispensed by individuals and corporations seeking to make money off of vulnerable people struggling with their weight. So, you might be asking, what makes me different? How did my 30-day diet lead to weight loss and positive cholesterol changes, while other similar diets led to weight gain and serious health problems and complications?

At the age of fifty, I have a physique and health level that surpasses that of many twenty and thirty-year-olds. I believe in the value of lifelong education, and I am currently pursuing a PhD in psychology after having received a bachelor's and master's degree in economics. I used many of the same skills that I gained in my academic career to study and analyze the scientific research pertaining to health, fitness, and weight loss, and in many instances, I have come away disappointed with the lack of practical strategies that have been developed to help ordinary people win their battles with obesity.

Like most of you, I am not employed in the fitness industry. I think my position as a fitness-industry outsider gives me a degree of credibility that many of the infomercial hucksters do not have.

Because I have a family and work full-time as an economist, I understand the impact that real life can have upon even the most well-intentioned diet and fitness plans. That is why I insist on a fitness framework that is realistic and incorporates a great deal of flexibility and adaptability.

Based on my knowledge and experience of the processes involved in weight loss and fitness, I was confident that I could not only maintain my level of fitness during the 30-day McDonald's diet, but that I could also lose some body fat along the way. Still, the overwhelming response that emerged as I went public with my plan reflected the oversimplified perspective that is so often put across in the media. It can't be done. He'll get fat. His cholesterol will skyrocket. He'll have to exercise all day long. These were only a few of the comments that some of the so-called experts were spewing before I started the diet.

The truth is, very few people take the time to properly educate themselves about diet and exercise, and fewer still actually apply these principles in their own lives. For the most part, the public's information about fitness, diet, and weight loss comes either from the marketing and advertising of those attempting to sell goods and services in order to make a profit, or from the media, which has a vested interest in making every subject overly simplistic or sensationalized.

I have said it before, and I will say it again: weight loss is straightforward. To achieve it and beat obesity, you simply have to make sure that you are taking in fewer calories than you are expending on a daily basis. On the other hand, if you consistently eat more calories than you need, *you will get fat*. It has little to do with carbohydrates, genetics, emotions, or any of the thousands of other tangential issues that the media and the weight loss industry tout as distractions. At its most fundamental level, weight loss is nothing more than a simple mathematical equation.

One of the most important tools that I used during the 30-day McDonald's diet was my ability to estimate the amount of calories that I needed to consume in order to maintain my weight, as well as the amount of calories that are in most of the foods that I eat. Twenty years ago, when I first began to take an interest in fitness, exercise, and nutrition, I did not know a calorie from a fat gram from a carbohydrate.

But I took it upon myself to learn about it, immersing myself in calorie-counting books and resources. Today, this information is freely available with a few clicks of the mouse on the Internet. Because I had not had any food from McDonald's for more than a decade before I started the 30-day diet, I spent some time researching the nutritional information and caloric content of many of their menu items prior to the beginning of the month-long process.

Using the information that is available to consumers for free on the McDonald's web site, I checked out the caloric content of all of the items of the menu. Based on these figures, I compared the caloric content of the McDonald's menu items to my own caloric requirements. My own needs require that I consume about 3500 calories a day. This figure is based on a number of factors, including my activity level. (Instructions for figuring out your own daily caloric requirements will be provided later in the book.)

Using this information, I was able to plan out my meals in advance with precision, ensuring that I would remain within the limits of my own caloric requirements. My plan was to eat 4 or 5 meals each day, with each meal providing about 800 calories. Based on my own understanding of the weight loss process, I knew that if I did not consume more than 3500 calories a day, I would not gain body fat. (When I talk about weight loss I do not mean body fat only. I will regard losing fat as losing only body fat. The difference is very important to understand. If you restrict your calories and do not exercise you will lose muscle and bone mass as well, and this will leave you flabby and unhealthy.)

I know what you are probably thinking: calorie-counting seems so out of sync with the currently popular beliefs about weight loss. Many of the most popular weight loss plans that are on the market today claim that calorie counting is unnecessary, claiming that if you stick to some other gimmick, such as monitoring portion sizes or eliminating carbohydrates, you will lose weight without having to count calories.

Well, these so-called "experts" are *lying* to you. While it is important to control portions, the very concept of portions is highly subjective and variable, and can change significantly from one restaurant or cook to another. Calories, in contrast, are consistent and reliable, and as such, are a much better basis for an effective weight loss plan. Once you have learned about calories and the caloric value of common foods, it's just like riding a bicycle: you'll never forget it.

After I had done some preliminary menu planning, I visited my physician to get some pre-diet health data and some lab work done so I could use this information as the starting benchmark for the 30-day diet. I explained my plan to my doctor, and like me, he was confident that the results would be just as I expected. My doctor shares many of my beliefs about health, nutrition, and fitness, in large part because I have helped him expand his knowledge base in these areas considerably over the years that we have known each other.

Okay, you may be thinking, I knew this guy was confident, but why would a doctor come to an economist for nutritional advice? Actually, I have helped several friends who are practicing physicians in this way. In the typical medical school curriculum, doctors-to-be receive less than thirty hours of instruction in nutrition. Even worse, they typically receive little or no instruction in exercise or exercise therapy. I find it to be very ironic that while the general public often regards physicians as the supreme authorities on health, nutrition, diet and exercise, medical students graduate largely uninformed about the major elements of health and fitness.

Following doctor's orders, I fasted the night before my blood work so that the laboratory technicians could get accurate results. After completing a thorough physical exam, I went to the lab, where a lab technician quickly filled three vials with my blood and placed a small circular Band-Aid over the red dot that marked the needle's insertion point. After being given an excellent bill of health, I was off to the first of the over 120 meals that I would eat at McDonald's during the next 30 days.

On the first day of the diet, I ate an Egg McMuffin; a McGriddle Sandwich with bacon, cheese, and egg; two coffees; a Big 'n Tasty with cheese; a small order of fries; three Diet Cokes; a Quarter Pounder; a 6-piece Chicken McNuggets; and a Chicken McGrill sandwich. In keeping with my plan, I spread this food out over four meals throughout the course of the day.

Throughout the first week of the diet, I was flooded with interview requests from national and international media outlets. Everyone I spoke with in the media wanted to know all-about the 30-day McDonald's diet and the effects it was going to have on me and, more specifically, my health.

I was amazed at and grateful for the vast interest that the project generated, but at the same time, I was shocked at the incorrect beliefs about diet, nutrition, health, and fitness that so many of the reporters, from both the United States and abroad, revealed in their questions. For example, it is widely believed that skipping meals is an integral component of weight loss. In reality, this is not true. An inadequate caloric intake can actually derail a weight loss effort, because it can trigger longstanding mechanisms in the human body that were developed to protect our prehistoric ancestors from periods of famine (we'll talk more about that later in the book).

If you only take one thing away from this book, I want it to be the ability to assess and evaluate claims about weight loss, diet, fitness, and exercise in an objective, rational manner. Critical thinking involves weighing the evidence and then using reasoning to make up your own mind about a claim, rather than relying solely on the assumptions and opinions of so-called experts on the subject.

During my early interactions with the media interviewing me about the diet, I marveled at the degree to which so many fundamentally wrong beliefs about diet and fitness have been cemented into the public consciousness over the years. The example that I used of meal-skipping as a part of the weight-loss process was a question that was put to me again and again in media interviews.

Using critical thinking and a basic level of knowledge about calories and caloric intake, it is easy to conclude that eating smaller meals throughout the day is an efficient means to achieve a lasting loss of body fat. However, this perception was not part of the weight-loss gospel that many media representatives had bought into, so they could not see the core rationality of the principles underlying the diet. Although I was grateful for the media attention to an issue that I believe needs more publicity, I began to feel like I was banging my head against the wall every time I had to defend my calorie-and-exercise-based approach to diet and fitness.

During the first five days of the McDonald's diet, I consumed 17,655 calories. Eating an average of 3,531 calories per day, solely from McDonald's fast-food menu, I lost 2 pounds of body fat. That's right—I lost 2 pounds! Even I was surprised when I saw these results. I had planned my menu choices in order to maintain my weight, so I was not expecting to post a weight loss. However, I did notice that my physique began to look more sharply-defined during the first five days of the diet.

Nothing else in my life had changed except for the food I was now eating; I was following my regular fitness regimen, averaging 1 hour and 15 minutes a day of aerobic and anaerobic exercise. In the process, I had lost 2 pounds of body fat, and I felt terrific. After the weight loss I experienced during the five days, I adjusted my eating plan by increasing my calories over the next couple of days. As a result, I began to consume a little more than 4,000 calories each day. I finished the first week with a daily average intake of 3,734 calories per day for a weekly total of 26,135 calories.

Week Two of the 30-day McDonald's diet started off with the news that my local gym gave us the go-ahead to film inside their facilities. I was filming all of my daily activities during the diet in order to accumulate footage for a documentary film of the process, which I titled "Down Size Me: Breaking the Fast-food Myth." Because I feel that exercise is such an important part of the weight-loss process, I wanted to make sure that the film included a substantial amount of exercise footage.

Although many fitness experts suggest that you can work exercise into your life using no equipment or small-scale equipment designed for home use, I am a big proponent of gyms and fitness centers as the core element of a fitness plan. These facilities provide beginning and long-time exercisers alike with both a space and an atmosphere that is motivational and highly conducive to developing and maintaining an effective fitness plan.

A misconception that is often held by the general public is that home exercise equipment can offer the same benefits as a gym membership. I affectionately call most home fitness equipment "closet equipment" because after a short period of use, it often goes into the closet, never to be seen again. Although effective exercising can be accomplished at home, I have witnessed very few individuals that possess the discipline to exercise at home consistently. There are far too many distractions in the home setting, and excuse after excuse will keep you from performing the activities that are necessary in order for you to achieve and maintain your fitness goals.

Many gyms and fitness centers offer a broad array of prepared exercise regimens. In many cases, individuals who are attempting to work out at home without the benefit of a planned exercise program misinterpret their activity level and end up overeating, gaining weight, becoming frustrated, and quitting altogether.

As an example, let's say you walk briskly for an hour around your neighborhood. During that time, you'll have burned about 200 calories, but now you think that since you've exercised, you can eat that 250-calorie donut that you've been craving. If you eat it, you've just added 50 calories of fat on your body. If you kept this habit up every day, you would have added at least 6 pounds of new fat on your body at the end of a single year.

Now, let's say you go to your local fitness center and perform a prepared exercise program for that same hour-long period. Based on an average of the energy expenditure that is required by these programs, you probably would have burned at least 500 calories. If you ate that donut now, you would be 250 calories in the negative. Repeat this pattern every day, and in the span of one year, you will have lost 26 pounds of body fat.

As I will emphasize throughout this book, the combination of exercise and your overall activity level is equally, if not more, important than the quality or type of food you consume. According to research published in the prestigious *Journal of the American Medical Association*, as many as 12 percent of the 2.1 million deaths that occur annually in the United States can be attributed to a lack of physical exercise. That means that as many as *250,000 deaths* each year could have been delayed or prevented if more Americans would make exercise an urgent priority in their everyday lives.

In addition, literally thousands of studies that have been conducted in recent years have shown that physical exercise has a significant impact upon our overall health and quality of life. Exercising regularly has been associated with substantial decreases in the risk of developing health conditions such as coronary heart disease, hypertension, cancer, diabetes, anxiety, and depression.

My regular exercise routine played an important role in determining the outcome of my 30-day McDonald's diet. Based on my calculations, the total number of calories that my body needed to function at rest (without exercise) was 2,080. Now, multiply that 2,080 by the first 13 days of the diet and the total amount of calories that my body needed at rest was 27,040.

However, during this period, I actually consumed 52,795 calories. That's an excess of 25,755 calories that my body would have stored as fat if I was not exercising during this period. In other words, I would have gained a little over 7 pounds of body fat in just 13 days! Yet, because I chose to make a little over an hour of exercise a part of my daily schedule, I actually lost 6 pounds of body fat in those first 13 days. I would say that exercise played an important role, wouldn't you?

The first day of Week Three of the diet happened to fall on April 15, 2004. It would end up being a late night for me, because I had put off finishing my income taxes until the deadline (Hey, nobody's perfect!). The following is an excerpt from my journal of that day:

> At 8:00 p.m., I paid a quick visit to a McDonald's by my office and found out that this one didn't take credit cards. I scrounged around my car for some change and found enough for a Double Cheeseburger off the Dollar Menu and a cup of water. I finally finished my taxes at 10:30 p.m. and had to then locate a post office that was open late. After dropping off my taxes I was still hungry, but alas, no McDonald's was open! I was doomed to starve throughout the night.

By 6:30 the next morning, I was off to McDonald's for a meal that consisted of a Sausage Biscuit Sandwich, a Hotcakes and Sausage Platter, a side order of scrambled eggs, and a large coffee, totaling 1,350 calories. I always emphasize the importance of being prepared, but I was not prepared with cash the night before. The most common downfall that can sabotage even the most well-intentioned diet, fitness, and weight loss plan is a lack of preparation for all possible contingencies and unforeseen circumstances.

In my own path towards fitness and health, I have always relied on the power of goals as a major source of motivation and discipline. Many people agree with the importance of goals, but often, they fail to develop specific objectives. In order to be effective, goals must be vividly envisioned, written down, and described with great accuracy and detail.

In addition, it is important to recognize that as circumstances change, goals must be able to be adjusted, as well. In order to ensure that your goals are always functional and relevant, you should revisit them on a regular basis and make any changes that will reflect your current situation and requirements.

At this point you are probably saying to yourself, "Yeah, yeah, I've heard it all before," and you are right. I know that even the lamest motivational speaker and most ill-advised diet "expert" can expound at length about the importance of goals. But if you look around you at the people who have achieved success, whether it is in business, personal relationships, or fitness, you will likely notice that all of these people share in common the fact that they devised a detailed, viable plan to achieve success and stuck to that plan. The more carefully laid-out a plan for achieving a goal is the greater the probability for reaching that goal.

Remember at the beginning of this chapter when I said that I knew beyond a shadow of doubt that I could not only stay fit eating McDonald's fast-food for thirty days, but that I could lose body fat along the way? Well, part of the reason for my success was that I vividly envisioned it, I wrote it down, and I allowed for adjustments if I wandered off course—and I was successful.

Once I mentally visualized what I would look like at the end of the 30 days, I wrote every detail down. I knew exactly what I would be eating at each meal and what each day's workout would entail; I did not leave anything open to chance. When I started to lose too much weight, I simply increased my calories to curtail the rate of weight loss. Conversely, if I would have started to gain some weight, I would have simply decreased my caloric intake. Making adjustments in order to stay on course is fundamental to the success of any goal. Every successful person that maintains a high level of health and fitness throughout their lives follows these principles.

During my early interviews about the diet, a comment I heard often was "You're not the average American," and you know what? They were right. According to health statistics, the average American is out of shape, overweight and/or obese. Taking those facts into consideration I definitely do not want to be the average American. Do you?

I watch about 5 hours of television per week and spend 9 hours per week training in the gym, for a total of 14 hours devoted to these actions each week. According to *The American Academy of Pediatrics* the average American child watches 28 hours of television per week, the average American male watches 29 hours of television per week, and a whopping 34 hours each week is devoted to television viewing in the life of the average American female.

Furthermore, the average American male, female, and child get little or no regular physical activity. Studies show that every two hours of television watching per day increases the risk of obesity by 23% and the risk of Type II diabetes by 14%. This is due to the commensurate decline in physical activity and increase in overeating that occurs in response to being inactive.

Television watching actually reduces your basal metabolic rate (the rate at which you burn calories) more than if you spent the same amount of time reading a book. In other words, you are burning more calories reading this book than if you were watching television. The health and fitness standards of the average American need to be improved, not accepted as normal.

The lifestyle of the average American involves little physical activity. As such, after 21 days of eating 88,415 calories of McDonald's fast-food as I did during the first three weeks of the diet, the average American would have gained approximately 13.5 pounds of body fat. According to the USDA, the average American adult requires roughly 2,000 calories per day, for 21 days that would total 42,000 calories. I guess I really *do* watch less television than the average American.

But who needs television when you're in Las Vegas? The beginning of Week Four found me under the bright lights of a city that has always set my soul on fire. I was visiting Las Vegas to attend the annual Electronics Transaction Association (ETA) convention. The annual convention is the industry get-together for those who, like me, work in the world of electronic commerce.

During the time I spent at the conference, I was not able to get to a gym for my daily workout. There are times when I am on vacation or away on a business trip that I may not be able to make it to the gym for my regular exercise routine. But just as I do not make a regular habit of overeating, I do not make skipping my workouts a regular habit.

I want to emphasize though, that at my level of fitness, I can easily afford to take a day or even a week off from training once in a while. However, if you are just starting out, you must understand that in order to reach your fitness goals there needs to be a specific level of commitment, dedication, and persistence before you even contemplate taking any time off.

As I mentioned before, the basic mechanics of health and fitness are simple: do not eat more calories than you expend. However, it's what I refer to as the "psychology behind the lifestyle" that ultimately determines whether an individual will achieve success in the struggle for improved health and fitness.

Your emotional and behavioral characteristics will form the foundation upon which you will build a healthy and fit lifestyle. If your mental and emotional foundations are weak before you undertake the daunting physical task of becoming healthy and fit, you will not achieve long-term results. My success with the 30-day McDonald's diet was determined well before I took the first bite of that McGriddle sandwich with bacon, cheese, and egg.

The psychology behind the lifestyle is a mindset, a way of thinking. It's about searching and discovering your true self. I was invited to attend a success seminar not too long ago, and one of the visualization techniques that were taught there was called "The Mirror Exercise." The exercise is a simple but powerful way to help people build self-confidence. It's designed to replace the negative, limiting thoughts that we often have about ourselves with a positive, self-affirming script.

Each night before you go to bed, stand in front of a mirror, by yourself, and demonstrate appreciation to yourself for all that you have accomplished during the course of the day. You start by looking into the mirror image of your eyes for a couple of minutes. Then start expressing appreciation to yourself, out loud, for any recent achievements that you accomplished, discipline that you displayed, or temptations that you withstood. This may sound ridiculous, but stay with me here.

You must maintain eye contact with yourself throughout the exercise. When you have completed appreciating yourself, end by saying "I love you." Maintain eye contact and feel the impact as though you are the one in the mirror listening to the appreciation. Do not cut yourself short; remember that this is an exercise geared to build self-confidence. And anyone who knows me well will tell you that I do not fall short in the self-confidence department.

For well over twenty years, I have been utilizing the mirror exercise on a daily basis, long before I knew it was called "the Mirror Exercise" and recommended by self-confidence experts. However, instead of doing it at night, I reverse the order and objective of the exercise by doing it in the morning and projecting the exercise onto the coming day.

I generally wake up at 4:15 a.m. and look at myself in the bathroom mirror. I critique my own physique and talk to myself about what I can do to improve it. During the diet, I could see my body changing almost daily. I would look at my abdominal muscles to make sure I was maintaining a "six-pack"; I would flex my arms in order to see the separation between my biceps and triceps, and I would examine the V-shape of my back. The mirror exercise really motivated me for my morning workouts.

I'm usually at the gym by 5:00 a.m. and on a stationary bike for my 20 daily minutes of aerobic exercise. Now, I make it a point to stay in what I call the fat-burning mode; that entails getting my heart rate up to where I would have a hard time carrying on a conversation with someone. I listen to upbeat music during my cardiovascular workout, but I never read or allow myself to become distracted by the hustle and bustle of the activity that is going on around me. Maintaining the link between the mind and the body is a very important element of maximizing your time in the gym.

After 20 minutes of aerobic activity, it's time for my anaerobic training (weight resistance) and no music. This is where the psychology behind the lifestyle becomes the most critical; I visualize every exercise before I ever touch the weight. With my mind focused on nothing but the exercise at hand, I start the course of action. As I begin to lower the weight, my lungs fill to capacity with air. I can feel every fiber within the muscle expanding with each repetition.

My heart pumps all the available blood to the area faster than the circulatory system can carry it away; the muscle becomes engorged with blood and swells to a noticeably larger size—this process is known as the "PUMP." The feeling is euphoric. I'm assisted on the last couple of repetitions by my training partner as I push the muscle beyond my mental limitations. You should understand that the body will do more than the mind will let it. Although I am exhausted, sweating, and drained of energy as my body starts the process of recuperating, I feel completely alive! After an incredible workout, I was once again off to McDonald's for my morning meal.

Day 26 of the diet represented the high point of my caloric intake during the month. I started it off with a Hotcakes and Sausage platter, a Sausage McGriddle Sandwich, two side orders of scrambled eggs, and a large black coffee. Throughout the course of the day, I also consumed a Double Cheeseburger, three Big Macs, a California Cobb Salad with Grilled Chicken, a McChicken sandwich, a small order of French fries, a hot fudge sundae, two baked apple pies, and a snack size Fruit 'n Yogurt Parfait for a total of 5,710 calories. Wow.

Throughout the 30-day diet, I was posting my daily journal and food intake on the web site of my non-profit organization, Truth In Fitness. On Day 28, I received an e-mail from a gentleman who was tracking my progress on the web site. He noted that I had not yet guzzled a Shamrock Shake, one of McDonald's seasonal specialty items. I replied that I would have one that day in order to fulfill my self-imposed requirement of eating everything on the McDonald's menu at least once.

To my surprise the McDonald's in my area were no longer making the Shamrock Shakes. However, having made a promise, I had to be sure that there were no Shamrock Shakes available. So I hopped in my car and drove to a few McDonald's in the surrounding area. Not finding any Shamrock Shakes, I took out my cell phone and called a few other franchises in the area. To my surprise, the McDonald's in Newport Beach reported that they were still offering Shamrock Shakes, so I drove over there lickety-split and indulged in one.

The 30th and final day of the diet started out with a flurry of interviews. One of the interviews was with a local newspaper *The Orange County Register*; they wanted to run a story in the next day's paper documenting the end of the 30-day McDonald's diet and announcing the free seminar that I would be holding on health and fitness that day.

During the interview, I was asked when I would have the results of my last blood test. I informed them that I would be having my blood tested on Monday morning, May 3, 2004, and the results should be in by Wednesday or Thursday of that week. After the interview, I considered the fact that the integrity of the project could be jeopardized by waiting two days before having my final blood tests. I immediately phoned my doctor's office and spoke with the head nurse, who was kind enough to make arrangements for me to come in that day and get my weight and blood pressure taken. (My official weight at the conclusion of the 30-day diet was a solid 214 pounds, which was 8 pounds less than my starting weight of 222 pounds.)

The nurse also arranged for my blood work to be done the next morning. I wanted to keep the integrity of the project as air-tight as possible, so until I received the results from my blood test, I continued to eat McDonald's food and nothing but McDonald's food in case eating something else would unduly influence the results of the tests. I had not come that far only to have the project's integrity questioned because of an accidental mix-up or error.

My last meal of the diet consisted of a Big Mac, a Double Cheeseburger, a 6-piece Chicken McNuggets, a snack size Fruit 'n Yogurt Parfait, and a medium Diet Coke. I had eaten more than 121 meals at McDonald's fast-food restaurants in the course of 30 days and lost 8 pounds of body fat, "Breaking the Fast-food Myth" in the process.

On the next day, May 1, 2004, I held a free public seminar on health and fitness. Eric Krondak, whom I helped to achieve his fitness goal earlier in the year, opened with his story.

The following are Eric's own words:

> Never realizing how fat I was getting, I eventually stayed away from the scale. When I started the program I was approximately 270 pounds; I've been even heavier at different times in my life. Even though I looked happy on the outside, I was not. It pained me having to buy larger pants (I was beyond a size 42 waist). I hated the way I looked; pictures of myself were difficult for me to view. I would diet and exercise for short periods, but never understood the difference between caloric intake and output. Therefore, I assumed since I exercised for five days I could eat whatever I wanted on Friday, Saturday and Sunday. Now when I look back, I realize that I took in somewhere around 5,000 to 8,000 calories each day.
>
> The hardest part of committing to a lifestyle change was thinking that I would have to give up all the foods that I love; pizza, In-N-Out Burgers, BJ's Pizzeria (especially the Pizookie cookies), cakes, popcorn, peanut M&M's, Mexican food, appetizers, etc. However, realizing

my health was at risk, my life had to be more important. I also had a deadline; I was getting married in 9 months. Not that I was doing it for the wedding, but at least it gave me a goal date.

In October I contacted Chazz and told him I wanted some information on working out. He suggested some routines and told me what my calorie intake should be. I followed his advice. I worked out on my own at our local clubhouse, and I noticed I lost some weight. This was a good thing. It gave me confidence and motivation to continue. I told Chazz I really wanted to lose weight, but with the holidays approaching and my family coming in from out of town, could we begin in January. Chazz understood and agreed.

On January 17th I started my exercise and nutrition plan. Chazz had given me a specific listing of foods and times to eat. He and I worked out together 6 days a week. After the first four days I thought I was going to die. He pushed me, but he knew my strength and how far I could go. After a month I noticed significant changes both in my strength and my weight.

By April I had lost 80 pounds and as of today (May 1, 2004) I have lost a total of 88 pounds. I feel terrific. I have more energy, more confidence, and a desire to live. I have received numerous compliments and have had people stop me to ask how I did it. I don't claim to be a spokesperson or expert, but I share my experience with them. Some people that I've spoken with have actually started or gone back to the gym and curbed their eating habits. The wedding is in a month, and I know I will look awesome. My fiancée

> and I are excited not only about our new life together but "my" new life.
>
> I'll never be able to repay Chazz for all he has done. He has never asked me for anything, except to be true to myself. Thank you, Chazz.

After Eric introduced me, I spoke on the fundamentals of health and fitness and then opened the floor up for questions. Holly, who was 54 years old and was holding 228 pounds on a 5'7" frame, raised her hand. You see, Holly had bought all the diet books, some closet equipment, and even went to a hypnotist in order to lose weight, but nothing had worked.

The following are Holly's own words:

> I met Chazz on May 1, 2004, at Triangle Square in Costa Mesa. I read in *The Orange County Register* that he would be discussing his 30-day adventure at McDonald's, and I thought it might be interesting to hear what he had to say.
>
> When Eric Krondak, the host for the event, told his story, it sounded like it was also my story. After seeing his "before" and "after" pictures I was hooked. I wanted to hear how he got to this point. He looked fantastic! Chazz came out to talk and seemed so *real*. But, I kept waiting for the punch line. There was no punch line, just truth. When he asked if anyone had any questions, I was hesitant to speak up. I guess I was afraid of getting laughed at, but I swallowed my pride and as my eyes teared up I asked, "How do you even start when you are this age, this overweight, and have multiple health problems?" Chazz looked me in the eyes, smiled and said, "Don't worry. It can be done if

you really want it bad enough. I will help you, but I won't do the work for you. Please stay and I will talk to you when this is over." I stayed and we have been talking ever since.

After six months, the results were undeniable. Holly's cardiovascular capacity increased tenfold, her knee pain had disappeared, and she experienced significant weight loss. Holly lost 51 pounds of body fat, not just weight loss. More important were the results from her blood work:

- Cholesterol (reference range 100-199): from a high of 231 down to 131
- LDL (bad cholesterol, reference range 0-129): from a high of 133 down to 52
- HDL (good cholesterol, reference range 40-59): from 52 to 57 (still within normal range)
- Triglycerides (reference range 0-149): from a high of 228 down to 88
- Mean Blood Glucose (reference range 95-110): from a high of 147 down to 120

Her doctor, having not seen her for six months, was completely surprised because he had been trying for years to get her to lose weight. He has since taken her off most of her medication and said that if she keeps this up, she should be able to stop all medication. She accomplished all of this by using very simple exercises that most people can do; no fad diets, just the willingness to work at changing her life.

Are you ready to change your life? Are you ready to become healthy and fit? In the following chapters, I will explain every step along the way to a healthier you. Health and fitness are subjective terms that have different meanings to different individuals, and as such, the principles that I outline will be able to be adapted specifically for your individual goals, and not in general terms. Whether you are male or female, young or old, looking to lose weight and slim down, gain muscle, or just become healthier, the principles are still the same. Know that I apply these same principles to everyday of my life. I don't just talk the talk—I walk the walk. Now, are *you* ready to stop talking and start walking?

How Did We Get So Fat?

As the rapid rise of obesity in the United States over the past several decades clearly indicates, a number of the defining characteristics of modern American society tend to promote the excessive consumption of the nutritional elements that can lead to unhealthy weight gain. First and foremost, many of the foods that are now widely available to American consumers are too densely packed with calories, causing many people to take in more calories than is necessary to maintain a healthy weight.

More specifically, recent scientific studies point out that foods high in fat, sugar, and salt, as well as an array of other chemicals and additives now comprise an unprecedented proportion of the American diet. The higher caloric content in the average American diet today compared to that which was common only a few decades ago is identified as one of the chief contributing factors in the emerging obesity epidemic that now plagues the country.

However, while the properties of many of the foods that are now represented in the diet of the average American tend to promote overconsumption, overweight, and obesity, the real source of the problem is the nature of the human metabolism. Simply put, our bodies are not properly equipped to deal with the nature and characteristics of the typical modern diet. The pace at which technology has developed in recent decades has far outpaced the human body's ability to adapt to changing conditions.

The Slow Pace of Evolution Versus the Rapid Advancement of Technology

The process by which humans (and, for that matter, all living organisms) adapt to changes in their environment is known as evolution. Evolution is a miraculous, complex process that has allowed the human race to survive and persist in an array of divergent conditions. However, the thousands of minute changes, mutations, and transitions that comprise evolution take place relatively slowly. Anthropologists and biologists typically measure the course of human evolution in units of thousands, or even millions, of years.

The twentieth century was characterized by technological change and advancement that occurred at a pace that was unprecedented in human history. When we think about the gains that were made in the course of the last hundred years, the first things that usually come to mind are single measures of material progress, such as the invention and distribution of the automobile or the developments of television and the personal computer. However, while these individual advances have all been significant, what is truly astounding is the degree to which together they have served to drastically alter the daily lives of average Americans.

With a few notable exceptions, the responsibilities and activities of most Americans today resemble those that were common one hundred years ago only in the broadest, most abstract sense. For example, while both early-twentieth-century Americans and early-twenty-first-century Americans typically start the day with breakfast, the effort and time involved in the preparation of food one hundred years ago far exceeds the few minutes of time and low effort involved in today's process of opening a container of yogurt, buying a bagel, or pouring milk over your favorite bowl of cereal.

Virtually all modern inhabitants of industrialized nations share a similar low-exertion lifestyle. The modern conveniences that define twenty-first century life may be expedient, but they have also served to force most of us into a comparatively sedentary way of life that is not conducive to optimal health, fitness, and well-being.

Because most modern men and women are, for the most part, largely sedentary, typically getting whatever physical activity that they engage in around the work place or home, scientists have long been challenged to analyze and understand the impact of our modern inactive lifestyle. However, researchers have recently been able to observe a community that represents many of the behaviors, habits, and tendencies, mirroring past generations. The Old Order Amish community, a highly insular religious group that eschews most modern conveniences and remains virtually unchanged from the way people lived 150 years ago, provided scientists with the perfect standard of comparison against which to examine and understand the broad, long-term implications of today's sedentary lifestyles.

The results of a multi-year investigation into the health, diet, daily physical exertion, and fitness levels of the Old Order Amish community were published in the January 2004 volume of the scholarly journal *Medicine & Science in Sports and Exercise*. The results of the study presented a truly remarkable window of insight into the consequences of the modern lifestyle and the transformative effects of a lifestyle that involves significant exercise and exertion.

Because the scope of the study was broad, the results that the researchers attained were too complex to detail specifically here. However, the overall gist of the findings revealed that a lack of exercise, rather than diet, is the chief cause of the obesity epidemic; which is a major health crisis facing the United States and in other nations today.

The researchers found that the members of the Old Order Amish community were largely traditionalists in their patterns of dietary intake. This means that their daily diet consisted of foods that are considered to be "bad" within today's popular nutritional culture—old favorites such as meat, potatoes, gravy, pancakes, breads, pies, and cakes, as well as many other dishes high in calories, fat, and refined sugar.

Despite the prevalence of this type of eating pattern, the researchers discovered extremely low incidences of obesity, high cholesterol, and type II diabetes, within the community. Among adult women, a very low rate of less than four percent were classified as obese; among adult men in the community, an astounding zero percent obesity rate was determined to exist by the researchers conducting the study. They explained that this low incidence of obesity was a result of the high levels of physical exertion required by the Amish on a daily basis. The study added strength to a 1981 study by Richard Hamman published in the American Journal of Epidemiology demonstrating that Amish communities are less likely candidates for heart disease due to lifestyle factors involving higher levels of physical activity. Without the convenience of modern devices, the Amish engage in a very high level of physical exertion, maintaining a near-ideal body weight while indulging on a diet high in calories, fat, and refined sugar.

The overall activities and responsibilities of daily life today for most people, however, are very different from the Old Order Amish community. While many Americans work long hours, growing numbers of them are engaged in white-collar work in the knowledge industry or service industry, labor that involves little physical exertion, and typically requires long hours sitting stationary behind a computer. While the *hours* that are worked by Americans today may be commensurate or greater than the schedules that were typical one hundred years ago, the degree of physical exertion involved in most Americans' daily lives has declined substantially at the same time that our caloric intake has increased.

Comparing twenty-first century life to life in the United States one hundred years ago yields a mind-boggling spectrum of differences. However, the points of divergence grow even more numerous if one expands the scope of the comparison and contrasts the lifestyle of the average twenty-first-century American with the lives of the humans that lived thousands of years ago.

For prehistoric humans, there was little time to devote to any other activity aside from the processes of hunting and gathering food. A great deal of effort was required to ensure that the adequate number of calories necessary to promote health and survival were consumed on a daily basis. Virtually every waking hour was invested in the process of seeking and preparing meat and gathering fruits, vegetables, and other sources of food.

In prehistoric times, only rudimentary forms of agriculture, horticulture, and food storage had been developed. As a result, the food available to humans was likely to vary considerably in terms of quantity and quality due to various external changes, such as seasonal differences, climatic shifts, famines, plagues, and other factors. Because of the inconsistency in the available food supply during prehistoric times, the processes of evolution worked to develop a number of physiological mechanisms that helped the human body survive through periods of scarcity. One of the most well-known mechanisms is the ability of the human body to extract and store energy from fats and carbohydrates.

While survival is a key objective of these mechanisms, reproduction is another important factor in the course that evolutionary changes take. As such, many of the mechanisms of the human body's ability to process food and store calories are meant to enhance and support reproductive success. This has particular significance for women and their struggles with weight loss, which will be discussed in greater detail later in the chapter.

As mentioned previously, the nature of evolutionary change dictates that it often involves thousands of years to be fully manifested in obvious adaptation in a species. When one considers the vast technological advances that have been made in only the last century, it becomes easier to understand why the demands of modern life and the capacity of prehistoric metabolisms are often incompatible.

This chapter will focus on an in-depth discussion of the body's metabolic processes, how they have developed throughout human history, what purposes they originally served and why they have contributed to the steep increase in overweight and obesity seen in recent years. In addition, we will begin to address the ways in which we can work with our admittedly old-fashioned metabolic processes in order to lose weight and maintain a healthy weight.

How Prehistoric Survival Mechanisms have Contributed to the Modern Obesity Epidemic

Even a casual glance at the newspaper can reveal the scope and severity of the obesity epidemic that is impacting the United States (and, increasingly, less developed counties such as India and Egypt) in the twenty-first century. It seems like every day, new scientific findings are released that reveal the nature and consequences of the growing spread of obesity among children, adolescents, and adults. The range of the negative side effects and detrimental health impacts that has come to be associated with obesity has also been expanded as a result of recent research.

At first, it may be difficult for us to understand why our bodies are adapted to process and store food in a way that can lead to obesity, which is a proven health hazard. However, when you compare the slow pace of evolutionary change to the extremely rapid rate at which technological advances have revolutionized agriculture, transportation, commerce, and food attainment and preparation over the last century, the reason becomes abundantly clear: modern technologies have outpaced the rate of human evolution. Our bodies employ food processing and storage mechanisms that were better suited to the days in which tribes of hunter-gatherers spent every waking hour engaged in the pursuit and preparation of foods, rather than the largely sedentary lifestyles we live today, in which we spend most of our time in stationary work, and making dinner involves no more effort than pulling into the fast-food drive-thru.

For vast stretches of human history, the possibility of obesity was negligible for most people. This was because the time and effort associated with attaining sustenance, paired with the inconsistent availability of food throughout the year, created a situation in which the over-consumption of calories was highly unlikely. Although famines, droughts, and food shortages continue to wreak havoc on populations in developing nations in the twenty-first century, food is available consistently and abundantly for the vast majority of Americans.

Feasts, Famines, and the Human Fat Cell

If you consider the workings of the natural world, it becomes readily apparent that seasonal changes, patterns of foliation and defoliation, and other factors all contribute to an inconsistent availability of food sources. As a result of these patterns that define the changes and cycles of the natural world, throughout vast stretches of human history, the food supply has been somewhat sporadic and inconsistent.

As technology has advanced, methods such as horticulture, agriculture, and food storage and preparation have been honed to a precise science. Today, food consumers notice hardly any difference in the availability of foods, regardless of the season. While particular types of foods may be limited in their availability or quality as a result of winter weather, drought, or other environmental changes, these instances are usually isolated, and have rarely, if ever, impacted the overall availability of an abundance of food choices for American consumers in recent years.

However, throughout most of human history, food availability was largely cyclical in nature. As a result, in order to ensure the survival and perpetuation of the species, human bodies long ago adapted the process of storing food energy in such a way as to sustain us through long periods during which food supplies may be limited.

When we read stories about prehistoric and ancient times, it is clear that social gatherings involving food were often a key component of human interaction in the past. To a large extent, these rituals have carried over into twenty-first century life. In the distant past, however, the cycle of feast and famine was a necessity that grew out of the lack of advanced food storage technologies.

In prehistoric or ancient times, feast rituals were often held in conjunction with harvest times, or in the aftermath of a major hunt. While part of the objective of these feasts was to celebrate the bounty of nature and give thanks for the success of the hunt or harvest, the more practical purpose of feasts in the ancient world was to prepare and consume a vast amount of food in a short time span.

Without the technological benefits of canning apparatuses, zipper freezer bags, and refrigerators, our ancient ancestors were often forced to feast whenever they were lucky enough to have gathered abundant food supplies. Although rudimentary food storage technologies were developed in the prehistoric and ancient eras, these techniques were often insufficient to store enough food to last through an entire period of low abundance.

Put simply, feasts were periods during which the ritual of overconsumption of food was encouraged. While the direct motivation of feasts likely varied in different social and cultural contexts, from a biological perspective, feasting involved eating amounts of food that were well in excess of the body's daily needs, leading to weight gain in the form of stored fat on the body. Later, during lean times, these fat stores could be used to sustain ancient humans when food was scarce.

While feasts are widely recognized as an important part of prehistoric and ancient societies, the opposite of feasting—periods of famine and food shortage—were an unavoidable part of life for much of human history. Although seasonal changes in the availability of fruits, vegetables, grains, and meats were the primary cause of periods of famine and food shortage, numerous other factors impacted the availability of food in the ancient world, as well.

Variables such as unexpected climate and environmental changes, war, human migration, population increases, species extinction, and the overuse of land all contributed to food shortages in ancient and prehistoric times. To a lesser extent, all of these variables continue to impact food supplies in developing nations today.

In industrialized nations, the advent of advanced technologies has allowed humans an unprecedented degree of control and stability in their food supply. However, due to the slow pace of evolutionary change, our bodies continue to process and store food energy as if our consumption was still governed by the uncertainty of the food supply and an inconsistent pattern of feasts and famines.

Human Evolution and the Processes of Metabolism and Body Fat Storage

From the perspective of twenty-first century Americans in the world's most prosperous industrialized nation, it is difficult to understand how the body's tendency to store food as excess fat could ever have been an evolutionary advantage. But if one thinks in terms of what types of traits would have been most likely to ensure survival and successful reproduction for prehistoric and ancient humans living with the inevitable fact of an inconsistent food supply, the ability to store food energy as fat for long periods of time could clearly be advantageous.

According to the research of anthropologists, famines and serious food shortages probably forced the excess fat stores of our distant human ancestors to be burned for energy once every three years, on average. The feast and famine cycle promoted weight gain during periods of food abundance, followed by weight loss during periods of food shortage. Overall, this likely resulted in weight equilibrium, with very little incidence of overweight or obesity, except among the most affluent individuals.

Because our bodies' metabolic functions were developed during periods of ongoing food shortages, one of the hallmark traits of the human fat cell is a stubborn resistance to shrinkage. Even throughout periods of increased physical exertion, minimized food intake, or both, the fat cell is often the last store of energy that the body wants to tap into. During the absences of physical exertion, muscles and organs will actually decrease in size before the fat cells are drawn on.

The landmark Dallas Bed Rest and Training Study of 1966, conducted mainly to help NASA scientists predict the effect of prolonged weightless space travel, had a profound effect on the medical community. Researchers at the University of Texas Southwestern Medical School confined five healthy, volunteered, twenty-year-old college men to bed for three weeks in order to measure their muscle loss and other factors. The researchers, testing the men before and after, found destructive physical changes that included a loss of muscle mass and a rise in body fat, as well as faster resting heart rates, higher systolic blood pressures, and a drop in the heart's maximum pumping capacity. These twenty-year-old men, in just three weeks of bed rest, developed physiological characteristics of men more than twice their age; however, the five men were able to recover and even surpass their original fitness levels after 8 weeks of exercise training.[1]

Thirty years later, in 1996, the researchers tested the same men again. The results were astonishing; the experience during three weeks of bed rest in their twenties had a more profound effect on their physical work capacity than did three decades of aging.[2]

Over the course of thousands of years, the human body has developed complex, intricate mechanisms and processes to deal with periods of food shortage. This development has been central to our survival and advancement as a species. Today, however, most Americans are faced with a surfeit of food. Still, our bodies remain mired in the period of ancient hunter-gatherers and require a certain amount of physical exertion.

The Prehistoric Origins and Modern Implications of Gender Differences in Fat Storage

As explored throughout this chapter, ancient and prehistoric times posed many challenges for humans. In addition to the overall unpredictability of the food supply, however, there were also unique challenges facing men and women.

Physiologically, male and female bodies diverge significantly, due in large part to their different roles in the reproductive process. These differences are the root of many other points of divergence in the male and female body, including differences in body shapes, musculature, and metabolic efficiency.

Both men and women have developed metabolic mechanisms that allow them to store fat when excess calories are consumed. However, because women are responsible for carrying unborn babies to term, their fat-storage and release mechanisms are more advanced and complicated than that of their male counterparts.

In a sense, all natural selection occurs with the end objective of increasing the success of the reproductive process. Biologists and anthropologists have confirmed that the way that fat tends to be stored and distributed on the female body is conducive to long-term storage and dispersal. This came about so that women may have a better chance at sustaining a nine-month period of pregnancy, even if the pregnancy occurs during a period of food shortage or nutritional scarcity.

Today, increasing numbers of women are returning to breastfeeding as a means of allowing their children to take advantage of the health benefits inherent in this natural food source. However, in the United States, most periods of breastfeeding continue for less than one year. In ancient and prehistoric times, however, nursing often extended throughout infancy and early childhood, requiring an even longer extension of the period during which the increased energy stores—garnered from either caloric intake or stored body fat—are needed.

Because women are theoretically able to become pregnant at any time during their child-bearing years, their bodies tend to store more fat and distribute it over a wider area than is typically seen in men, in case the pregnancy occurs during a famine or a food shortage. This explains why women, in general, have a higher percentage of body fat than men do. It also explains why women's body fat tends to be dispersed over a wider area, with the greatest concentration in the hips, buttocks, and thighs: this wider distribution allows for efficient mobility and a longer depletion time in the case of a food shortage.

With men, excess body weight tends to be stored in the form of fat concentrated in the abdominal area. There are advantages and disadvantages to this archetypally "masculine" pattern of weight gain. (Some women also tend to gain weight in this pattern, especially those who have entered menopause.) Because the weight is concentrated in a smaller area, it is often easier to stimulate the release of the excess fat through reduced calorie intake and an exercise regimen. This explains why men often outpace their female counterparts in weight loss efforts.

However, the main disadvantage that has been associated with the typical male pattern of abdominal weight gain is a higher degree of general health risk. Although the source of this heightened risk remains unclear, some scientists have speculated that it is a result of the close proximity of excess body fat to the vital organs that are enclosed in the abdominal and chest cavities. By contrast, the female pattern of weight gain in the hips, thighs, and buttocks largely evades the body's major organ systems.

Further extending the analysis of the reproductive association with body fat, it has been found that a healthy level of stored fat actually increases the reproductive success of women. Adolescents and young adults whose body weight falls within the normal range are more likely to experience the onset of menstruation in a timely manner.

In contrast, adolescents and young adults who, for whatever reason, have fallen below the level considered to be a healthy body fat often have delayed onset of menstruation or highly irregular menstrual cycles. For example, young female athletes engaging in rigorous, sustained training sometimes experience irregularities or interruptions in their menstrual cycles.

This stands as further evidence that, from an evolutionary standpoint, stored fat is beneficial to successful reproduction, particularly among females. Because a significant amount of stored fat is necessary, from an evolutionary position, to ensure the success of a pregnancy and after-birth care and feeding, much of women's metabolic activity is geared towards storing fat, particularly during the child-bearing years.

Because of the efficiency in fat storage that has been developed as a core component of the metabolism of the human female over millions of years, the process of weight loss can prove to be frustrating, particularly for women. When initiating a weight loss program, a period of time must often elapse before a woman can convince her body to begin releasing its fat stores.

Due to the inherent metabolic resistance that is part of the female metabolism, this is sometimes a time-consuming experience, and male weight-loss partners may quickly exceed their female counterparts in total pounds lost. However, because the process of weight loss ultimately boils down to eating fewer calories than you exert in energy expenditures, your efforts will be rewarded in time.

The Evolutionary Origins of Human Taste and Food Preferences

In the previous section of this chapter, we discussed the ways in which the human body has developed a complex, intricate system for processing and storing food energy as fat. This was necessary because of the food scarcity, famine, and unpredictability that often characterized the environments of our prehistoric and ancient ancestors.

The frequency of food shortages throughout human history has impacted evolution in a number of other ways, as well. One of the most interesting fields of research to emerge over the last several decades comprises the studies that have attempted to trace the origins of human taste preferences. Just as our bodies have adapted to store food energy in the most efficient manner possible, our taste buds have evolved to ensure that we are predisposed to choose the foods that will tend to promote the most reproductive success, and in this manner, ensure the perpetuation of the human race.

However, as I pointed out in the previous discussion, the pace of evolutionary change is exceedingly slow. During the millions of years that it took to develop advantageous taste preferences that appealed to humans and ensured that we would make beneficial, health-promoting food choices, many environmental and technological advances and transformations have also occurred, particularly over the course of the last century.

Just as our fat storage mechanisms are geared toward the times in which tribes of hunter-gatherers roamed the Earth, our taste preferences are geared toward maximizing caloric and fat intake. These inherent preferences were developed during the millions of years when food sources were somewhat scarcer than the aisles and aisles of abundance you can find at the local supermarket.

As we will discuss in detail within the chapter on calories, fat has a caloric value more than double that of carbohydrates or proteins. From an evolutionary perspective, then, eating high-fat foods would be the most efficient way to ensure that humans were consuming a sufficient number of calories. In this context, it makes perfect sense that we have a seemingly boundless appetite for high-fat foods, or foods that smell, taste, or feel like they have a high fat content.

In prehistoric times, if a human found a high-fat food, it would be beneficial, from an evolutionary standpoint if they consumed a substantial amount of the food. In this manner, over the course of millions of years, natural selection ensured that the humans who were successful in reproduction were more likely to have a preference for high-fat foods.

In the past, this preference was beneficial, because high-fat foods were few and far between in the prehistoric environment. Today, however, they are plentiful and easy to obtain. So, twenty-first century Americans remain saddled with the vestiges of a once-beneficial craving for high-fat foods in the midst of an unprecedented period of abundance of these foods.

The longstanding scarcity that helped to select this trait as an advantageous strategy for survival is largely a thing of the past. As a result, the human craving for high-fat food has become, as scientists term it, *maladaptive*. That means that the high-fat taste preference not only serves no clear purpose in the modern environment, but that it has also begun to be actively detrimental to the human population, as evidenced by the fact that as many as two-thirds of the adult population in the United States is overweight or obese.

Researchers have posited a similar pattern of development for our lingering sugar cravings. From an evolutionary perspective, it is thought that the prehistoric sweet tooth was an inducement to eat ripe fruit when it was available. Not only does ripe fruit have a wide array of nutritional benefits, but it also has a high concentration of sugar, which can serve as a source of energy in the short-term.

However, our residual sugar cravings have lingered long past their evolutionary shelf life. Today, in spite of the best efforts of the nation's nutritionists, most Americans do not consume a quantity that even comes close to achieving the recommended daily servings of fruit. Still, like the lingering preference for high-fat foods, the sweetness preference has remained intact.

Today, it is more likely to be fulfilled with the consumption of highly-processed snack foods than ripe fruit. While the over-consumption of calories and fat are typically identified as the chief sources of the current obesity epidemic, many nutritionists assert that it is likely no coincidence that obesity became a massive problem during the same century that saw the first processes developed for the mass refinement of sugar.

Aligning Our Stone-Age Metabolisms with the Realities of a Fast-Food World

Now that we have gained some insight about the evolutionary origins of our taste preferences and the processes that our bodies use to store food energy as fat, is it possible to devise some middle way, a compromise that calls a truce between our prehistoric genes and the twenty-first century? It definitely is! All that it takes is some planning and consideration.

There has been a lot said in the media in recent years about the evils of the modern diet, and to a large extent, I agree with these criticisms. But, at the same time, I believe that we are all thinking beings that are each ultimately responsible for the decisions that we make and the food that we choose to consume. Now that you know some of the prehistoric origins of your overwhelming desire for candy bars or a thick T-bone steak, I hope that it will be a little easier for you to acknowledge your cravings, but then re-direct that urge towards a comparable food choice that is more beneficial for your overall health.

I believe that we are at an important crossroad in our society. For the first time in recent memory, fast-food restaurants are incorporating a wide array of fresh food selections into their menus, and these changes are being rewarded with substantial sales. This trend is allowing American consumers to make healthier food choices in a convenient format that more closely matches the pace of our modern lives.

The process of evolution and change that has occurred over millions of years is nothing short of miraculous. These minute shifts and transformations have allowed humans to survive and thrive as a species. While the technological advances and resulting lifestyle changes that have occurred over the course of the last century are amazing, they have also served to broaden the gap between the workings of our bodies and the modern environment.

In addition to the mysterious workings of our metabolisms, digestive systems, and weight regulation processes, humans are blessed with a degree of intelligence and a capacity for self-reflection that is unmatched in the animal kingdom. Although our food cravings and urges can feel overwhelming and overpowering at times—particularly during periods of high stress—we must exercise our power of rational thought to work through the often-contradictory messages that our bodies are sending us.

Although technology has swept twenty-first century Americans into lifestyles that were scarcely imaginable one hundred years ago, it is our responsibility to exercise restraint and use the unprecedented knowledge, tools, and resources we have access to and devise a compromise between our health and our cravings. Acknowledging and working to modulate the prehistoric origins of our often unhealthy eating patterns and taste preferences represents a strong step in the right direction.

Calories: Understanding the "Math" of Weight Loss

One of the paradoxes surrounding modern American life can be seen in the fact that even as we are, collectively, more overweight than at any other time in history, vast segments of the population—as many as fifty million people at any given time—consider themselves to be following a weight reduction plan or diet. For many Americans, dieting has become a way of life.

How can this be? How can the prevalence of obesity and overweight have attained epidemic proportions during the same period in which the diet industry has grown into an economic sector that is responsible for more than fifty billion dollars of revenue annually?

The Rise of the Fad Diet and the Diet Industry

Throughout the twentieth century, myriad fad diets and "magic" weight loss regimens have been developed and popularized, with each trend usually evaporating from the public's awareness as rapidly as they were first embraced. However, as the prevalence of overweight and obesity has attained epidemic consequences over the course of the last several decades, the number and influence of "fad" diets have increased significantly.

Although diet books have been available for decades, the past few years have seen a broader spectrum of diet regimens entering into the marketplace and, for a short time, capturing the interest of a greater consumer base. The most recent of these diet plans include the South Beach Diet, Dr. Atkins' New Diet Revolution, Body for Life, the Zone Diet, Slim-Fast, Dr. Phil's Ultimate Weight Solution, the Grapefruit Diet, the Cabbage Soup Diet, and the Hollywood Miracle Diet, as well as innumerable others that have not attained the same degree of nationwide prominence.

Each of these popular diet plans offers its own unique approach to weight loss. The Atkins diet advocates the use of an unbalanced, protein-heavy eating regimen that eliminates most, if not all, starches and sugars. The Slim-Fast plan and the Hollywood Miracle Diet both rely on modified fasting and liquid meal replacement, a strategy that nutritionists caution is difficult to sustain in the long-term.

The Grapefruit Diet, the Cabbage Soup Diet, and other similar regimens rely excessively on the consumption of a single food, which is not conducive to the balanced eating that facilitates a healthy lifestyle and sustainable weight loss. While Dr. Phil's Ultimate Weight Loss Solution seems to advocate a more sensible low-calorie, high-fiber approach; however it relies too much on the use of processed products, supplements, and meal replacement products to be considered genuinely healthy.

What Do All of These Diets Have in Common?

Despite the extreme divergence that characterizes the rules and methods that define many of the top weight-loss regimens today, there are a number of key similarities that all of these popular diets share. The most notable similarity is that none of these diets have been proven to help people maintain weight loss in the long-term. Indeed, based on recent studies, most of these diet plans have been shown to have an abysmal success rate, with the number of individuals who lose weight keeping it off in the long-term only about 3% of the time.

The release of The Zone Diet program is an example of an approach that is too complex to be sustainable in the long term. In order to adhere to the strictures of the regimen, dieters are expected to carry out complex mathematical calculations in order to ensure that their meals will keep them in "the zone." Does this sound like something you're willing to do while getting dinner together on a busy weeknight?

In addition, like many other recently released diets, The Zone is marketed with an array of heavily processed, market-ready nutrition bars, meal replacements, and other products. In my experience, the more a diet expects you to buy and eat pre-packaged specialty products, the less likely you will be able to work it into your lifestyle in the long-term.

Another similarity that many of today's most popular diets share is the fact that style, rather than substance, is their chief source of appeal. The age of epidemic obesity in the United States has dovetailed with the age of mass media advertising, and as a result, the diet industry has at its disposal a vast arsenal of tools and tricks that it skillfully deploys to exploit the increasingly desperate population of overweight and obese Americans.

Television, radio, print, and Internet advertisements, late-night infomercials, product placement, and celebrity endorsements—all of these tools serve to entice American consumers struggling with obesity. These tools are extraordinarily effective, prompting Americans to enrich the diet industry to the tune of more than fifty billion dollars annually.

Sometimes, the claims that the diet industry makes are so exaggerated as to border on sheer falsehoods. For example, the Body for Life program claims that you can drastically alter the appearance of your body over the course of a 12-week program. While this remarkable claim may prove accurate if you happen to be an out of shape athlete who has taken months off from his or her training program, it is almost guaranteed to be false if you are a normal person with an out-of-shape physique that is the accumulated result of years of neglect, under-exertion, and questionable eating habits.

In other cases, diet plans rely heavily on the advertising power of the media to gain credibility and popularity. Perhaps no other diet plan has taken to this approach with more success than the South Beach Diet. Essentially a modified Atkins-like plan, the South Beach Diet attained astounding popularity through the use of a number of skillful cross-promotional campaigns.

Initially, the plan itself derives from the originator's collaboration with several up-market Miami-area restaurants. In addition, food industry giant Kraft licensed the name of the diet in order to release a series of heavily-processed, pre-packaged diet foods and meals. Both of these clever promotional plans reveal more about the business shrewdness of the cardiologist who developed the diet than its ability to sustain long-term weight loss.

I can think of virtually no other industry that reaps as much profit from such an unproven, ineffective range of product offerings, can you? The two key ingredients that make this extraordinarily unfounded degree of profitability possible is the desperate difficulty that many Americans have with losing weight and maintaining a healthy weight, as well as widespread misunderstandings about the way that the weight loss process works.

The Rise and Fall of Calorie Counting

In the earlier decades of the twentieth century, most weight loss regimens were based on strictly regulating caloric intake. However, in recent years, the emphasis on counting calories has diminished to some degree. Most Americans today who are attempting to lose weight do not rely on calorie counting as a major component of their diet strategy. Indeed, many of the most popular fad diets, such as the Atkins plan, imply that calories are ultimately unimportant in the weight loss process.

THIS IS SIMPLY UNTRUE. In the process of weight loss, the number of calories that are consumed is the single most important factor. While there are many other factors and variables that will also impact the success and effectiveness of a weight loss effort, caloric intake is the key deciding factor that will determine 1) WHETHER you will lose, gain, or maintain your weight and 2) HOW MUCH weight you will lose or gain.

In order to understand the way that food calories impact the weight loss process, it is crucial to gain a basic understanding of what a "calorie" is and does. In this chapter, we will explore the concept of calories and discuss the ways that changing your caloric intake can impact your weight.

What is a Calorie?

In the discussion of diets and weight loss, calories are often mentioned as if they were a nutritional unit. However, this is not the case. In fact, a calorie is actually a measurement of energy and energy potential. Even non-food items can be measured in terms of their caloric content, because a "calorie" is simply the amount of energy that a particular substance can produce.

Specifically, a single calorie represents the amount of energy it takes to increase the temperature of 1 gram of water to 1 degree Celsius, or 1.8 degrees Fahrenheit. To use a non-food example that shows the way that calories measure energy potential, one gallon of gasoline contains approximately 31,000 calories. So if your car could run on McDonald's fare it would take about 52 Big Macs to go the same distance as it would be able to travel on a single gallon of gasoline.

Think of your body as a miraculous machine that contains a number of distinct, but inter-related systems. Energy is needed to power the hundreds of processes and functions that your body is carrying out every second of the day in order to sustain your life. Even if you expend very little energy every day in exercise or movement, your body still requires a significant amount of energy to power functions such as breathing, maintaining your heartbeat, moving blood through your veins, processing the solid food and liquids that you consume, and conveying nutrients throughout your body.

Food Calories: Quantity vs. Quality

In the general terms of assessing how much energy potential a certain substance has, you could say that all calories are created equal. However, when we use the concept of calories to talk about the energy values of different foods, you will find that not all calories are created equal, especially when you are strategically selecting a diet that will maximize your weight loss potential.

The most crucial distinction between different types of foods in terms of caloric values can be seen in the fact that carbohydrates and proteins possess only four calories per gram, while fats have nine calories per gram. This five-calorie discrepancy may not seem like much, but when you are trying to plan a healthy, filling menu, the calorie difference between fats, proteins, and carbohydrates quickly becomes apparent.

For example, a single tablespoon of olive oil—which is comprised of pure fat—contains 120 calories. Clearly, a meal that consisted of nothing more than a single tablespoon of olive oil would not be very filling, satisfying, or appealing. At the same time, for the same caloric value, you could eat one-fourth of a pound of white meat chicken.

Based on this example, the basic philosophy to wisely budget your daily caloric intake in order to get the best "value" for your food choices begins to be revealed. Do you think that one tablespoon of olive oil or one-fourth pound of white meat chicken would be the better choice as the foundation for a healthy, satisfying meal?

The Role of Calories in Weight Gain and Weight Loss

Now we have begun to see the way that different food choices can have decidedly different impacts in terms of caloric intake. But where do these numbers fit in to the overall process of weight loss?

As I mentioned earlier in this chapter, calories measure energy potential in food. In your body, the energy units that are measured in calories are used up and "burned" as part of the ongoing function of the metabolism. In this way, the energy potential that you take in when you consume food is transformed by your body into a kind of fuel that can be used to power processes such as moving, breathing, and other functions.

The metabolic process is complex, and it can be impacted by a number of internal and external factors and variables. Basically, your metabolism transforms the carbohydrates in the solids and liquids you have consumed into glucose. In much the same way, fats that have been consumed are rendered as glycerol by the metabolic process, and proteins are turned into amino acids.

These three processes, for the most part, are responsible for transforming all of the foods that you consume into the raw materials that your body needs to carry out the functions that are needed to sustain your survival. Glucose, glycerol, and amino acids are all vital components of human health and nutrition.

If one consumes too few carbohydrates, proteins, or fats, the body is unable to produce the needed levels of glucose, glycerol, and amino acids, and a potentially dangerous nutritional deficit can occur. On the other hand, if one consumes more calories (carbohydrates, fats, or proteins) than the body needs to carry out its functions, other types of unhealthy nutritional balances could be the result.

Indeed, the consumption of a number of calories that far exceeds the body's energy needs is the chief cause of the overweight and obesity levels that have reached epidemic proportions in modern American society. Calories that are consumed in excess of the body's energy needs are stored as fat.

Therefore, they cannot be stored as amino acids—for the body, fat is the preferred mode of storage. When you consume too many calories, beyond the carbohydrates stored as glycogen in the liver and muscles, the excess is transformed into fat cells. When the equivalent of 3,500 excess calories has been consumed, this surplus will be manifested as one pound of body fat. Over time, this kind of consistent over-consumption of calories will inevitably result in the accumulation of excess body fat, which, in turn, often leads individuals to the unhealthy weight levels that can be classified as overweight or obese.

Lasting Weight Loss: Psychology or Math?

In the diet literature that is produced by the fifty billion dollar weight loss industry, hundreds of reasons are set forth as the cause of overweight and obesity in the United States. In recent years, for example, the prevalence of the Atkins diet has convinced many that excess sugars and carbohydrates in the diet are solely responsible for obesity.

In my view, much of today's diet literature is emotionally manipulative and allows many dieters to be comforted by being provided an outside target to blame for their predicament. Many recent books, programs, and systems give the impression to focus more on the emotional and social aspects of obesity rather than personal responsibility. As an example, Bob Green's "Make the Connection" program, which achieved widespread popularity in the mid-1990s through Oprah Winfrey, placed great emphasis on emotional exploration during the process of weight loss.

I don't deny that social, emotional, and psychological issues sometimes contribute to weight gain. Indeed, I think that these types of problems often greatly contribute to the excess consumption of food and calories that is the chief cause of obesity.

As a result, I often encourage people seeking to lose weight and maintain their weight loss to explore some of the emotional and social components of their eating habits. This is particularly important in order to ensure that those individuals who have successfully lost weight will not immediately return to their previous patterns of consistent over-consumption after their weight loss goals have been achieved.

However, even though I acknowledge the validity of exploring the emotional and social facets of overeating and weight gain, I also remind those considering weight loss that the same principles of excess caloric consumption that can facilitate the accumulation of body fat and weight gain can also result in weight loss if they are applied in reverse. Simply put, while 3,500 excess calories will result in a gain of one pound of body fat, you can take solace in the fact that the reverse is also true: If you expend 3,500 more calories than you consume, you will necessarily and inevitably lose one pound of accumulated body fat.

It is not complex. It's physics. It's math. Let me say it again: *If you expend 3,500 more calories than you consume, you lose one pound of accumulated body fat.* Rather than focusing all of your efforts and energies on searching out the deep-seated emotional causes and psychological roots of your excess weight, it is more productive to focus on what science has revealed as the mathematical inevitability of weight loss if more calories are burned than are consumed. If you follow this principle, *you will lose weight.*

Think of calorie consumption and weight gain as a chemical equation. If you think back to the days of high school chemistry, physics, or biology, you probably remember that there are some principles that are referred to as "constants." These principles, sometimes expressed in the form of mathematical equations, are always true, no matter what the circumstances.

The principle that expending 3,500 calories more than you consumed will result in a pound of weight loss is just this sort of bedrock, scientific fact. For a very small number of people, other health factors may impede the weight loss process.

However, for the vast majority of individuals, the key to lasting weight loss is ensuring that you are consuming calories and burning calories at a level that will result in an ongoing calorie deficit. As we have learned in our discussion of calories, we know that the total quantity of an individual's caloric intake can be determined by looking at both their consumption of food and their expenditure of energy. If it were one of those mathematical equations that I mentioned above, it might be shown as something like this:

calories from food and beverage intake – calories used for energy
= net calories consumed

Simple enough, right? Using this formula and the knowledge that it takes a net deficit of 3,500 calories to equal one pound of weight loss, it will be fairly easy for you to determine the amount of calories that you will have to consume and how much exercise that you will have to do to ensure that you will lose weight.

However, there is one important variable that is not strictly defined in this equation, and that is determining how many calories that you require for your basic energy needs. This number is not the same for everyone; to the contrary, it varies significantly according to each person's weight, height, age, and gender.

Before you can make an accurate assessment of your nutritional and exercise needs in a weight loss plan, you must determine what your caloric intake requirements are, based on your current weight, height, age, and gender data. The best way to do this is by employing a proven caloric-intake formula. One of the most popular and trusted of these formulas is known as the Harris-Benedict formula. Simply plug your personal data into the appropriate equation, and the answer will be a close estimate of your daily caloric intake requirements.

For Adult Males:

66 + (6.3 x body weight in pounds) + (12.9 x height in inches) - (6.8 x age in years) = targeted daily caloric intake

For Adult Females:

655 + (4.3 x weight in pounds) + (4.7 x height in inches) - (4.7 x age in years) = targeted daily caloric intake

The figure that these equations will produce is the number of calories per day that your body needs to maintain healthy functioning and processes. This figure is known as your *basal metabolic rate*. However, the Harris-Benedict equation outlined above does not take into consideration the level of extra physical exertion that you may be engaging in. Using the figures attained from the previous equation as a starting point, you can employ the following extended equation to account for various levels of physical activity. If you encounter any difficulty using this formula, please use the online calculators that are available in the "useful tools" section of the truthinfitness.org web site. Here, by simply plugging your personal weight, height, and age data, caloric needs will be estimated automatically.

Activity Multiplier (can be used for both men and women)

- If you are sedentary (little or no exercise, office job), multiply your basal metabolic rate by 1.2
- If you are slightly active (light exercise/sports 1-3 days per week), multiply your basal metabolic rate by 1.375
- If you are moderately active (moderate exercise/sports 3-5 days per week), multiply your basal metabolic rate by 1.55
- If you engage in heavy exercise (hard exercise/sports 6-7 days per week) multiply your basal metabolic rate by 1.725

Using these equations and the resulting figures, you have been able to attain a good estimate of your basic caloric needs. Keeping in mind the key concept that a net deficit of 3,500 calories is needed to result in the weight loss of one pound, you can begin to devise a weight loss strategy that combines sound nutrition and increased physical activity. By manipulating these two variables, each individual who is seeking to lose weight can develop their own personalized approach, combining a calorie-reduction plan and an exercise regimen that is realistic and yet still sufficiently rigorous to ensure ongoing weight loss.

Achieving a Calorie Deficit with Smart Food Choices and Exercise

The key to successful weight loss is ensuring that through a combination of reduced caloric intake and increased energy expenditure, you are creating a calorie deficit. As mentioned, you will need to create a deficit of at least 3,500 calories to lose one pound of stored body fat. The average weekly loss of body fat that occurs during a targeted, effective weight loss effort ranges from one to three pounds. To achieve a loss in this range on a weekly basis, you will have to plan your nutritional intake and caloric expenditure, using your basal metabolic rate as a basis for comparison, to ensure that you have achieved a calorie deficit of 3,500 to 10,500.

Initially, you may believe that this sounds like a daunting task, particularly if you have ever looked over a chart of the average calories that are expended doing common exercises. Here are a few common activities and their average levels of calorie expenditures per hour:

Sleeping	55
Sewing	85
Eating	85
Sitting	85
Knitting	85
Standing	100
Driving	110
Office Work	140
Housework, moderate	160+
Golf, with trolley	180
Golf, without trolley	240
Gardening, planting	250
Dancing, ballroom	260
Walking, 3mph	280

Table Tennis	290
Gardening, hoeing etc.	350
Tennis	350+
Water Aerobics	400
Dancing, aerobic	420+
Skating	420+
Aerobics	450+
Bicycling, moderate	450+
Jogging, 5mph	500
Gardening, vigorous	500
Swimming, active	500+
Cross country ski machine	500+
Hiking	500+
Step Aerobics	550+
Rowing	550+
Power Walking	600+
Cycling, studio	650
Squash	650+
Skipping with rope	700+
Running	700+

Don't get discouraged! Remember, you are not going to rely upon exercise alone to create the level of calorie deficit that you need to lose weight. Instead you are going to strategically combine reduced caloric intake with increased physical expenditure to achieve the calorie deficit that you need to ensure a steady, safe weight loss rate of one to three pounds a week.

Are you thinking that this sounds impossible? Have you had bad experiences in the past with bland, unappealing reduced-calorie foods? Well, times have changed a lot in recent years, and many of the highly-processed, nutritionally suspect foods that were marketed by the diet industry in the 1970s, 1980s, and 1990s are no longer regarded to be the ideal option for those who are seeking to achieve lasting weight loss.

Instead, today's calorie-restricted weight loss regimens are more likely to emphasize fresh, unprocessed foods prepared in a simple but appealing manner. Below is an example of a healthy menu that would provide about 1500 calories.

Breakfast

- Two eggs, scrambled
- Light whole grain toast with light margarine
- 8 ounces skim or 1% milk

Morning Snack

- Orange slices or sliced celery

Lunch

- Sandwich assembled using turkey or ham, light wheat bread, and lettuce, cucumber, and tomato
- Carrot and celery sticks
- Sliced kiwi fruit
- Iced tea or skim or 1% milk

Afternoon Snack

- Nachos, made using low-fat baked tortilla chips and fat-free salsa

Dinner

- Stir-fry with shrimp, broccoli, and bell peppers over 1 cup brown rice
- Chinese cabbage vinaigrette salad (1 tsp. oil and seasoned rice vinegar)

Dessert

- Frozen grapes served over one cup of low-fat or fat-free vanilla yogurt

---

Doesn't sound too bad, does it? If this type of menu is used as a guideline every day and paired with regular physical exertion such as daily vigorous training, it is virtually guaranteed that an ongoing weekly weight loss ranging from about one to three pounds could be achieved and maintained.

When people who are struggling with their weight contemplate making a change to a healthy lifestyle, they often feel discouraged, because in the human imagination, even small changes in habits can seem like a formidable undertaking. However, in my experience, when the prospect of a major life change is broken down into its small, constituent parts, the possibility of making and maintaining healthy lifestyle changes becomes much less threatening.

As demonstrated in this chapter, a menu that reflects the dreaded calorie restrictions that are a necessary component of lasting, effective weight loss need not mean that you will feel deprived, hungry, or unsatisfied. Indeed, most dietitians strongly recommend that even the strictest reduced-calorie diets must include variety, appeal, and aesthetic interest in order to ensure that individuals embarking on the challenge of weight loss will not be discouraged.

With this weight-loss program, I want to take this idea even further. Modern life is hectic in a way that few of us would have been able to predict even twenty years ago, and the preparation of a fresh, wholesome, reduced-calorie meal is not always possible or appealing in all circumstances.

For this reason, this program will give you strategies that will carry your determination to lose weight and make healthy food choices with you into the "real world." I realize that real life isn't always the utopia of boundless food choices, limitless preparation time, and compliant family members that some dieticians seem to believe that it is. It is my mission to give you the viable tools and strategies that you will need to focus on making positive food choices in a wide variety of situations and circumstances.

With these tools and strategies, I am confident that you will be equipped to maintain the calorie deficit that you need to lose weight no matter where you find yourself, even if a hectic after-work schedule and family obligations have found you ready to turn dinner responsibilities over to McDonald's or Burger King. As I said earlier in this chapter, the mathematical equation that states that a 3,500 calorie deficit is necessary to lose one pound of stored body fat is a scientific constant. That means that the equation applies whether you are eating a fresh, wholesome, home-prepared dinner, or whether you are forced in a pinch to opt for a fast-food salad.

Don't get me wrong; I am not making the case that you should eat fast-food for every meal and expect to lose weight and maximize your health. However, the point that I am trying to make is that there are usually a range of both good and bad food choices everywhere that we look. Armed with an understanding of the crucial role that calories play in the weight loss process, the personalized caloric intake that your weight, height, age, and gender dictates, and the strong determination to maintain the necessary caloric deficit, you can navigate any eating situation successfully.

All that you need to do to ensure your success in this program is to take the time to do a little research about the food offerings and general nutritional values that are available in the stores, restaurants, and other eating establishments that you typically frequent. I hope that the prospect of "research" doesn't scare you off—it may sound harder than it actually is.

If you have Internet access from your home or office, you can quickly and painlessly get access to detailed nutritional information for virtually all the menu items served at the major fast-food chains. As the

Internet becomes a more important business tool, many regional and local establishments are also beginning to employ this platform as a way of distributing nutritional information, as well.

If Internet-based nutritional information is not available, ask for a pamphlet or brochure stating nutritional facts from your favorite restaurants (most chains are likely to have these available upon request). As an alternative resource, use a generic calorie-counting calculator or reference guide to make a rough guess as to the caloric content of your favorite dishes.

Many of the more recent calorie-counting guides that have been published in book form also offer guidelines for estimating portion sizes by describing visual comparisons, such as the little-known fact that a single serving of meat should typically be the same size as the palm of your hand (not counting the fingers or thumb). Once you gain a working knowledge of common calorie counts and portion sizes, you will be well equipped to navigate any dining experience successfully, while remaining in alignment with your targeted weight loss goals and caloric deficit objectives.

I know from my own past experiences, as well as my encounters with others who are struggling with weight loss, that the prospect of major change can be disheartening. Now that you have a better understanding of the "math" of weight loss, use this knowledge to remind yourself that if you diligently do your part and stick to the targets set forth in the equations presented in this chapter, lasting weight loss is guaranteed.

Aerobic and Anaerobic Activities

In our discussion concerning the evolution of obesity throughout human history, we learned that technology and rapidly changing lifestyles have caused a major imbalance for many people living today. Although we still have pretty much the same energy requirements, musculature, taste preferences, and fat-storing capabilities as our prehistoric ancestors living tens of thousands of years ago, we live in a vastly modernized environment in which food is plentiful and easily accessible while most work involves little or no physical labor.

In our discussion of calories, we learned that by making a number of relatively minor, deliberate manipulations to our caloric intake, we could jump start the weight loss process. Weight loss, is, fundamentally, a physical process that inevitably occurs when a number of conditions are met. The foolproof formula of consuming fewer calories while expending more calories is the only time-tested approach that has been shown consistently to help people just like you achieve lasting weight loss.

Throughout this book, I have made it clear that developing and sticking to an exercise plan is a major component of weight loss. If you are serious about moving towards physical fitness and improved health, you have to commit to making exercise a part of your life. Any diet plan that promises weight loss without requiring regular physical activity is offering little more than false hope.

Aerobic and Anaerobic Exercise: A Primer

So far, I've generally used the term "exercise" without making distinctions about the different types of exercise. Although there are literally hundreds of physical activities that you can engage in as part of your weight loss journey, all of these activities can be classified as one of two types of exercise: aerobic or anaerobic.

Aerobic exercise is the kind of exertion that involves the rapid movement of your larger muscle groups, such as your arms, legs, and hips. This type of exercise increases your heart rate, quickens your pace of breathing, and heightens the level of oxygen in your bloodstream. All of these changes help contribute to weight loss.[3]

While aerobic exercise has come to be the most common form of exercise associated with weight loss, recent research has begun to identify the importance of anaerobic exercise in the process, as well. *Anaerobic* exercise is, in some ways, the opposite of aerobic exercise, in that it does not involve extended, continuous activity.

Some of the most common forms of anaerobic exercise include weight lifting, push-ups, pull-ups, isometrics, calisthenics, and toning exercises. Literally translated, the term "anaerobic" means "without air." This does not mean that you are supposed to hold your breath while you are lifting weights; to the contrary, proper breathing while performing anaerobic exercise is vital in order to ensure that your body is getting the full benefit of the activity.

However, what "anaerobic" *does* mean is that this kind of exercise does not produce the same sustained changes in heart rate, breathing pace, and blood-oxygen levels that aerobic exercise does. Instead, anaerobic exercise helps your body primarily by increasing strength, power, and performance through the muscles. Furthermore, during the process of losing weight, engaging in anaerobic exercises such as weight-lifting helps by increasing the efficiency and speed of your metabolism.[4]

In essence, this type of exercise makes your body a more efficient fat-burning machine. Fitter, more muscular bodies tend to burn fat faster and more effectively than do overweight, untoned bodes. As such, anaerobic exercise can actually speed up the weight loss process by increasing the speed and efficiency of your metabolism.

The ideal exercise plan for maximizing weight loss will combine both aerobic and anaerobic activity.[5] These two types of exercise are complementary to one another. If you think about it from an evolutionary point of view, our prehistoric ancestors were not just undertaking chores that were comparable to either jogging *or* lifting weights; instead, their typical daily activities included tasks that involved both aerobic and anaerobic exercise.

Since one of your major objectives in the weight loss process is to overcome the long-outdated limitations of our human metabolism, the most advantageous approach to take in designing an exercise plan is seeking to mimic the kind of combination of activities that were part of daily life for our distant ancestors. This will involve both aerobic and anaerobic exercise.

If you combine the benefits of aerobic and anaerobic exercise in a sensible, challenging and consistent routine, your quest towards fitness, health, and weight loss will be significantly expedited.[6] I asked you to think of calories and formulating your ideal caloric intake as the *math* of weight loss. It may be helpful for you to think of an exercise plan that combines aerobic and anaerobic activity as the *engine* of weight loss.

In the chapter in which we discussed calories and optimal caloric intake, I told you that the figure that you had to take into consideration when calculating your target food consumption during weight loss was your *basal metabolic rate*. From a mathematical perspective, this figure is a "given" that remains stable. However, from a real-world fitness perspective, your basal metabolic rate can and will change, making the weight loss process that much easier.

What's the catch? Well, in order to take advantage of the ability to manipulate your basal metabolic rate, you must commit to an exercise plan, ideally, one that combines the best of both worlds: aerobic and anaerobic exercise.

You may be thinking that that sounds easier than it actually is. It may be one thing to agree that an exercise program is important while you are snuggled in your favorite recliner reading this book, but it's another thing to actually get up early in the morning and trudge to the treadmill or stair climber and translate that abstract idea into real, tangible, sweaty motion.

I have a theory that it is part of human nature to avoid exercise at all costs. Now, I have no scientific proof to back that up, but considering what the experts say about the complex ways that our taste preferences and metabolisms evolved over thousands of years, it also makes sense to me that we would have inherited an inexplicable urge to avoid exertion (and thus save precious energy) until we are faced with a serious, unavoidable threat.

For our prehistoric ancestors, the presence of a life-threatening hazard may have frequently taken the form of a hungry saber-toothed tiger or a rampaging wooly mammoth. For us modern humans, the looming threat takes a much different, less immediately threatening shape. It may even look just like your favorite, well-worn recliner, with a bag of potato chips and the remote control within easy reach. However, if we do not respond to this threat by using exercise in the same way that our ancestors used exertion to escape danger, the consequence is likely to be the same as it was thousands of years ago: a significantly reduced span of life.

I know it is hard to commit to and follow through with a regular exercise program. In spite of my natural reluctance (which I think everyone, no matter what their fitness level, has to work through), I make the decision to do something positive for my health and my life. I make the decision on a daily basis. Instead of reaching for the snooze button two or three times, I make the conscious, deliberate decision to use my short time on Earth in a beneficial way and I *exercise.*

Part of my dedication to fitness is the result of my own motivation, something that must be cultivated by each of us individually. In another chapter, you and I will together tackle the challenge of developing and sustaining the high level of motivation that is a universal characteristic of people who have successfully lost weight and made the journey from obesity to excellent health and physical fitness.

However, if you are like me, you may need to understand the need for something on a rational level before you can make an emotional investment in the follow-through. I understand this approach to decision-making completely, and in truth, I feel like it is very important to understand and commit to major undertakings on both an intellectual and an emotional level in order to ensure success.

In the remainder of this chapter, I am going to discuss the basic components and characteristics of aerobic and anaerobic exercise. Many diet plans may vaguely direct you to engage in regular exercise, without explaining in detail the "why" and the "how" factors. I want you to understand completely the "why" and the "how" factors of aerobic and anaerobic exercise, so that you can fall back on the rational justification for exercise when your emotional motivation may falter in the midst of your own personal journey towards weight loss and fitness.

For both aerobic and anaerobic exercise, I am going to outline the ways that these activities promote health, fitness, and weight loss. In addition, I am going to provide some basic guidelines that will help you devise a uniquely-tailored exercise program that will substantially improve your body's ability to burn fat and lose weight effectively and efficiently.

Aerobic Exercise

Although the processes and mechanisms that the human body uses to create and distribute energy are multi-faceted and complex, the single most important role is that which is fulfilled by oxygen. We all know that we cannot live without adequate oxygen supplies, but sometimes people do not realize that even a seemingly small decline in the oxygen levels in the bloodstream can lead to the energy imbalances that tend to initiate catastrophic medical events, such as strokes and heart attacks. In order to ensure that the body operates properly and that all bodily functions can be maintained, a constant, stable supply of oxygen must be available.

When we avoid regular exercise and fall into a sedentary lifestyle, the body's ability to create and distribute oxygen throughout the body effectively gradually diminishes. Conversely, when we engage in a regular exercise program, particularly one that emphasizes both aerobic and anaerobic activities, we can actually improve and expand the body's ability to distribute oxygen in an efficient, effective, and health-enhancing manner.[7]

Basically, an activity that involves the sustained, repetitive motion of your larger muscle groups can be categorized as aerobic exercise. When we engage in this type of exercise, we ensure that the muscles are receiving a sufficient supply of oxygen. As a result, this oxygen can be used to create energy in the process that is known as aerobic energy production.

As your level of aerobic fitness increases over time, your heart and blood flow will also increase in efficiency. At higher levels of fitness, more oxygen will be delivered to the muscles in a shorter period of time. It is by this process that the complex measure of fitness that is sometimes labeled "stamina" will be able to increase. Highly efficient oxygen delivery allows you to exercise longer and harder, and this in turn allows more fat to be burned.[8]

From a scientific point of view, the increased production of energy from oxygen stores is the most significant outcome of aerobic activity. However, from a broader perspective, there is a wide spectrum of consequences that result from this primary process, and all of them are beneficial for those seeking to lose weight, improve their health, and move toward excellent physical fitness.[9]

Although it may seem as if the idea of using aerobic activity to improve your health and lose weight has been around forever, in truth, it was first widely advanced in the 1970s, which roughly corresponds to the advent of the jogging craze. Over the course of the last several decades, scientists have delved deeply into the challenge of exploring physical fitness. As a result, we now have a much fuller understanding of the health and fitness benefits that are associated with aerobic exercise.[10]

Many people whose health and fitness levels have begun to suffer in recent years often seek a "magic pill" that will improve their health, increase their quality of life, and reverse their slide into obesity. Well, the "magic pill" won't be found on one of those late-night infomercials. If you are looking for the answer to a wide array of health problems, aerobic activity appears to be as close to a "magic pill" as anything that I have encountered.

Improved Heart Health and Cardiovascular Function

Regular aerobic exercise has been demonstrated to directly affect cardiovascular health. Scientists have found that individuals who engage consistently in aerobic exercise can drastically improve the functioning of their heart, as well as their entire cardiovascular system. In some cases, aerobic exercise can even reverse existing cardiovascular damage and decline.[11]

This finding has major implications for everybody, but it is particularly important for those with cardiovascular disease, heart problems, or a family history of either of these problems. Considering that these conditions are some of the most significant health problems facing Americans today, the ability of aerobic conditioning to minimize risk and reduce the severity of cardiovascular problems is an important breakthrough.[12]

Cholesterol Levels

Recent research has also identified the ways in which regular aerobic exercise can have a positive effect on the body's level of cholesterol. High cholesterol content that is a defining characteristic of many of the foods containing saturated fat are available in modern grocery stores and restaurants, resulting in a nationwide epidemic of excessive bloodstream cholesterol levels that has emerged in recent years.

High blood cholesterol has been linked with a number of health problems, including, most importantly, heart disease. Aerobic exercise has come to be recognized as one of the most effective strategies to reduce the unhealthy type of cholesterol and promote the healthy type of cholesterol.[13]

HDL cholesterol has come to be known as the "good" cholesterol, because scientists have found that it contributes to cardiovascular health by promoting the free, unobstructed flow of blood through the arteries. Regular aerobic exercise has been linked in research with increased levels of HDL cholesterol.

On the other hand, LDL cholesterol is typically regarded as "bad" cholesterol. This is the fatty substance that is often responsible for the clogged arteries that can lead to impaired oxygen delivery to the heart and heart disease. However, these levels tend to drop among individuals who are engaging in regular aerobic exercise.

Reduced Health Risks

Among those who engage regularly in aerobic exercise, the risk of developing many common health problems has been found to be significantly reduced.[14] Problems and conditions including hypertension, heart disease, heart attack, stroke, and diabetes have all been shown to be minimized when a consistent program including aerobic activity is followed.[15]

Taken together, these health problems represent some of the most common, costly, and potential lethal medical issues that are currently challenging the American population. From a health perspective, taking on the commitment of regular aerobic exercise can drastically improve your overall well-being and quality of life, as well as limiting your expenditures for health care related to these common problems.[16]

Quality of Life Improvements

Improved health and increased physical fitness are probably two of the most significant immediately effective ways to improve your level of happiness and satisfaction, as well as the overall quality of your life. However, in addition to the health and medical benefits that researchers have linked to regular physical exercise, recent studies have also associated a dizzying array of other factors that help you feel better when you are engaging in a consistent sensible aerobic exercise program.

Some of the variables that have been shown to improve when people are engaging in regular aerobic exercise include reduced stress, anxiety, and depression. Sleep can improve, as can sexual performance and satisfaction. Chronic fatigue and lethargy tend to fade, and energy levels increase. Chronic pain can lessen.[17]

Regular aerobic exercise can also positively impact the course of aging, as well. Research has shown that individuals who engage in regular aerobic exercise fare much better during the aging process than their sedentary counterparts. The ease of mobility, the onset of diminished cognitive functioning, and the ability to live independently have all been shown to be impacted positively by aerobic exercise.[18]

I don't mean to position aerobic exercise as the solution to every problem that you face. Unfortunately, there are many issues in life that cannot be worked out on the treadmill. But these are all findings that have appeared in the most respected scientific journals over the last several decades. Taken together, they present a pretty compelling case for making the commitment to regular exercise, don't you think?

Implications for Weight Loss

I saved the best for last. Of course, if you have read this chapter to this point, you already know that aerobic exercise helps you lose weight. But I may not have emphasized enough that regular aerobic exercise can help you lose weight quicker, more effectively, and more permanently than dieting alone.[19] When you produce energy and heighten oxygen levels by engaging in aerobic exercise regularly, you are honing your body's willingness and ability to release fat stores, resulting in weight loss.[20]

So, the next time that you are huffing and puffing on the elliptical machine, think of it this way: you are not only burning fat at that moment. At the same time that you are burning fat today, you are also making an investment, if you will, in your body's ability to burn fat better and more efficiently tomorrow. In this way, your commitment to aerobic exercise exponentially increases the success of your weight loss effort.[21]

If getting bored is your concern, it shouldn't be: there is a broad spectrum of potential aerobic activities for people of every skill level and interest. I have encountered individuals who have had success using a variety of activities as their primary aerobic exercise. Examples include:

- Walking
- Hiking
- Aerobic dance
- Swimming
- Rollerblading
- Bicycling
- Rowing
- Cross-country skiing
- Jogging
- Running
- Dancing
- Stair climbing
- Aquatic exercise classes
- Elliptical training

There is something for everyone, and if you really crave variety, you can devise a fitness plan that encompasses a number of different aerobic activities.

More Science

Still not convinced as to the importance of aerobic exercise? Need still more logic and data? Well, let's explore the scientific processes that are involved in aerobic exercise a little more so you can better understand the science, chemistry, and biological processes that you initiate when you are engaging in this kind of exertion.

The Cardiovascular System

The term "cardiovascular" refers to the system and organs that are involved in the movement and distribution of blood and oxygen throughout the body. As the name implies, the heart and the veins, arteries, and capillaries are the major component of the cardiovascular system.

The heart acts as the engine of the cardiovascular system, providing the motion and energy that moves blood and oxygen throughout the body. The network of veins, arteries, and capillaries act as the infrastructure through which these vital substances are transported, in a role that is something like the interstate highway system of the body.

The respiratory system is also closely related to the role of the cardiovascular system, particularly in relation to the movement of oxygen in the bloodstream. Although breathing through the mouth and/or nose is typically regarded as respiration, the more crucial aspects of the respiratory system have to do with the transfer of oxygen to the body's many organs, tissues, and systems through the blood vessels. Just as important is the movement out of carbon dioxide at the conclusion of the respiratory cycle.

Nutrients from consumed food, as well as oxygen, are carried to the cells in the blood. Once delivered, they are used to create energy for muscle movement. However, if more nutrients are delivered than movement is required (for example if you are eating a pint of double-fudge ice cream while doing nothing more challenging than lounging on the couch all day long), these nutrients will be stored as fat, rather than transformed into the chemicals that can later be burned for energy in muscle movement and contraction.[22]

Another major function of the cardiovascular system is the removal of toxins and byproducts. After the process of creating energy has been completed, several substances and byproducts, including carbon dioxide, water, and lactic acid, must be carried out of the body, or to different locations, where they are expelled or put to additional use.

When you engage in an activity that requires a short burst of energy, your body uses anaerobic energy production to power the motion. This process draws upon the stores of energy that remain within the muscular tissue. Typically, this is glucose, a simple sugar. There are many health benefits of anaerobic exercise (which will be discussed in detail later in the chapter), but the process of building cardiovascular strength occurs primarily during exercise that is sustained for longer periods of time.

When you exercise for a sustained duration, your body requires increased levels of oxygen consumption to maintain your performance. It is in this situation that the aerobic energy production processes kick in. Although this process uses some glucose as a fuel, it also initiates the use of stored body fat as a fuel.[23]

When increased oxygen levels are needed in order to sustain long-term aerobic activity, the short-term supplies that are stored in muscular tissue are no longer sufficient. Instead, after several minutes of sustained aerobic activity, the body begins to dip into the reserves of stored body fat to find fuel to burn in order to meet the increased oxygen requirements of this type of exertion. As such, this is the juncture at which meaningful weight loss begins to occur, and it explains why aerobic exercise is an indispensable component of the weight loss process.[24]

When you first begin engaging in aerobic exercise, it will not take very long for you to experience a feeling of fatigue that will probably threaten your ability to continue at the same level of exertion for very long. However, once you have made aerobic exercise a regular feature of your daily schedule, your stamina will increase considerably, allowing you to endure aerobic activity for longer periods of time.

This, in turn, will allow you to spend more time burning stored body fat, and thus, lose more weight. In addition, over time, your body will become more efficient in the process of delivering both oxygen and stored body fat to be used as fuel during the aerobic exercise process.[25] This will serve to increase the efficiency of your metabolism. To return to the metaphor that I used earlier in this chapter, it will make your body a more effective, efficient, harder-working fat-burning machine.

Mapping Out Your Zone: Maximum and Target Heart Rate *More Science*

In order to maximize your body's efficiency in the process of fat-burning, you need to ensure that your exercise activity remains within a range of exertion that will optimize the fat-burning process. One way to do this is to calculate your target heart rate, using one of several common formulas. In order to calculate your maximum heart rate, which is needed in several of these formulas, do the following equation:

Maximum heart rate = 220 - age

Now, using the figure that you derived, use one of the following equations to calculate your target heart rate for aerobic exercise. This is called the Zoladz method, and it is based on the work of renowned exercise physiologist J.A. Zoladz.

Target Heart Rate 1 = Max Heart Rate - 50 beats
Target Heart Rate 2 = Max Heart Rate - 40 beats
Target Heart Rate 3 = Max Heart Rate - 30 beats
Target Heart Rate 4 = Max Heart Rate - 20 beats
Target Heart Rate 5 = Max Heart Rate - 10 beats

The figures that you arrive at using these equations should give you a fairly accurate estimate of the zone you want to remain in during aerobic exercise in order to ensure that you are optimizing your fat-burning capability. The first number, Target Heart Rate 1, represents your target heart rate during the initial or early phase of working out, such as a warm-up.

On the other hand, the last number, Target Heart Rate 5, represents exercise that is so vigorous that only professional athletes reach it on a normal basis. Most beginning exercisers find a comfortable, but challenging pace between levels 2 and 3. As you progress on your path towards increased physical fitness, you may find that you have to increase your exertion in order to achieve this heart rate.

Generally, experts suggest that you aim to work at about 50-85% of your maximum heart rate in order to achieve optimal aerobic conditioning.[26] However, it is important to note that this is a range that should be interpreted differently for each individual. Furthermore, a physician or an exercise physiologist should be consulted if a more in-depth analysis of your situation is required.

If you are not convinced about the physical, mental, and weight loss benefits of aerobic exercise, you're a hard sell! Although there is a lot of compelling evidence that demonstrates the advantages of aerobic exercise, the ideal approach to fitness combines both aerobic and anaerobic exercise.[27]

Actually, in my personal philosophy of fitness, aerobic exercise and anaerobic exercise are like two pieces of a puzzle, complementing one another perfectly. You will maximize your body's ability to lose weight and burn fat if you combine both of these elements in your fitness program. In the next section, I will talk a little about the importance of anaerobic exercise.

Anaerobic Exercise

As I mentioned before, "anaerobic" literally means "without air." The lack of air that this name is referring to is related to the absence of the oxygen-increasing properties of aerobic exercise. Despite what their names imply, anaerobic and aerobic exercises are complementary parts of the fitness process that each serves to maximize the effectiveness of the other.

By definition, anaerobic activity takes place in short bursts. In order to be defined as true anaerobic activity, a single session of anaerobic exercise cannot last long enough to activate the body's long-term energy production process. However, many short repetitions of anaerobic exercises can be completed in one session.[28]

In the preceding discussion of aerobic exercise, we focused primarily on the fat-burning potential of that type of activity. Because it takes long-term durations of aerobic exercise to activate this process, anaerobic exercise does not burn fat. However, it can help you to achieve a number of other, desirable health and fitness objectives that aerobic exercise alone cannot.

The process that occurs when anaerobic activities are being performed involves the rapid transformation of existing supplies of glucose into lactic acid and adenosine tri-phosphate (ATP). This process is known as anaerobic glycolysis, or more commonly, as anaerobic metabolism.[29]

When the anaerobic metabolism process is initiated, the accumulated lack of oxygen, as well as the build-up of lactic acid, results in a phenomenon known as an oxygen debt. In order to achieve a degree of equilibrium in the body's major systems, a rapid intake of oxygen is necessary. This is achieved through the heavy, labored breathing that often can be observed in the aftermath of anaerobic exercise.

Lactic acid, which is one of the byproducts of anaerobic metabolism, is the substance that is responsible for the burning sensation and rapid-onset muscle fatigue that is one of the hallmarks of anaerobic exercise. In the past, this sensation likely alerted our prehistoric and ancient ancestors that the muscle system being used had nearly reached the limit of its exertion. Today, for savvy exercisers, this sensation signals one of the vital characteristics of muscle-building activities.[30]

In the short-term, engaging in anaerobic activities can increase your strength and endurance and increase the conditioned appearance of your body, which can often go a long way towards boosting the outward changes that are apparent during the weight loss process. In the long-term, engaging regular anaerobic activity can actually serve to increase the efficiency of your metabolism.[31]

There are a number of benefits associated with a more efficient metabolism. Most significantly, the rate at which you will be able to lose weight will speed up substantially. As I told you in the chapter about calories, your basal metabolic rate (the number of calories that you burn when you are at rest) typically remains stable.

However, after engaging in an exercise program that includes anaerobic activity, your basal metabolic rate will increase due to added muscle mass. This means that your body will burn calories and fat at a higher rate. Also, it means that you will be able to consume a greater number of calories without gaining weight.

Other Benefits of Anaerobic Exercise

The last several decades have yielded an array of astounding research results pertaining to the benefits of anaerobic exercise, resistance training, and strength training. In the years immediately following the discovery of the health and weight-loss benefits of aerobic activities, an inordinate amount of research focus was centered on identifying and communicating the benefits and advantages associated with regular participation in anaerobic exercise.

During this period, strength training, resistance training, toning exercises, and calisthenics were somewhat marginalized, thriving only among small communities of fitness hobbyists. However, in the 1980s and 1990s, research efforts began to extol the benefits of a fitness regimen that combined elements of both aerobic activity and anaerobic exercise.[32]

In the years since, additional studies have identified a wide array of health and fitness benefits associated with many popular anaerobic activities. These health benefits are in addition to the most commonly cited positive outcomes of anaerobic exercise, namely, increased strength and endurance and a more efficient metabolism.

Safer Sports and Exercise Participation

Although it may seem counter-intuitive, many people, especially athletes, engage in anaerobic exercise as a way of reducing their risk of injury in other types of sports and exercise. Studies have shown that individuals who regularly exercise anaerobically have much stronger muscles and joints than their counterparts.[33]

This difference can prove to be the decisive factor in avoiding injury, particularly in high-exertion exercise, such as running, or contact sports such as football.[34] However, even for fitness enthusiasts (or aspiring fitness enthusiasts) who are not professional athletes, the safety gains associated with anaerobic exercise can be substantial.

On a related note, anaerobic exercise has also been linked to better balance and stability. This can be beneficial for all individuals, but gains in this area may be particularly helpful for elderly individuals, or any person whose balance and stability is impacted by health conditions or other problems.[35]

Another application for anaerobic exercise that was first identified in the sports world is injury rehabilitation. Over the past several decades, the practice of treating injuries with mild, targeted anaerobic exercises has gained widespread prevalence.[36] This approach is best supervised by a trained physician or exercise physiologist, but it does attest to the restorative power of anaerobic activity.

One of the most intriguing areas of research that has begun to be explored in recent years is the use of anaerobic exercises with middle-aged and elderly individuals. Although we commonly associate elderly people, in particular, with muscular weakness and increasing frailty, researchers have demonstrated that moderate periods of regular anaerobic activity can significantly lessen the effects of the aging process.[37]

One major finding has shown that anaerobic exercise, especially strength training, can substantially diminish, and in many cases even reverse, the bone loss that is often a component of the aging process.[38] Both bone density and brittleness can be improved, reversed, and prevented with targeted strength training programs, eliminating a major source of health problems and quality of life issues for elderly women and men.[39]

Another health issue that has been shown to be affected by anaerobic exercise is heart disease. As I reported earlier in this chapter, heart disease is the leading cause of death in the United States, and its treatment costs patients and taxpayers billions of dollars annually.

Recent studies have gathered promising results, however, indicating that strength training and other types of anaerobic exercise has been shown to reduce the risk of heart disease and limit its severity in patients already diagnosed with the condition. Also, strength training was found to have a similarly beneficial impact upon hypertension and the reduction of bad cholesterol.

Now, let's talk about some superficial reasons for anaerobic exercise. Put plainly, anaerobic activity can significantly change your appearance, probably faster than you ever dreamed possible. While aerobic activity is more efficient for losing body fat, it commonly takes a little longer for this type of exercise to make a noticeable difference in the way that you look.

Because of the unique nature of anaerobic activity, however, and the special processes that it initiates in the body, the results from consistent, ongoing anaerobic exercise are often dramatic. While aerobic activity results in broad weight loss, the targeted toning capability of anaerobic activity often results in more recognition of your efforts and the changes you have made.

I joked earlier about superficiality, but in truth, I don't think that you should discount the powerful motivation that you can derive from making noticeable changes in your outward appearance. All too frequently, people who have experienced obesity for a long span of time suffer from low self-esteem and a lack of confidence.

The striking differences in the way that these individuals often look and feel a short time after taking up an exercise routine that involves both aerobic and anaerobic activity has a profound impact on virtually every aspect of the way that they experience life and relate to other people. It's amazing; I have often compared it to a flower coming into bloom.

For older people, particularly, anaerobic activity can significantly change appearances. The gradual sagging that we all associate with older men and women is actually a slackening of the musculature that is known as atrophy.[40]

Contrary to what you have probably been told all of your life, *it is not inevitable.* This radical change in appearance can be diminished considerably. If you engage in regular strength and resistance training, you will not experience the physical impact of aging upon your appearance to the same degree that your unfit peers will. At the risk of sounding arrogant, I think that my own physique is incontrovertible proof that the aging process can be drastically slowed down with a strategically developed, sensible fitness plan that encompasses both aerobic and anaerobic elements.

Pulling it All Together

I hope that I have conveyed to you the health benefits and weight loss advantages that can be attained through the development and consistent use of an exercise regimen. While I feel that it is important to devise a realistic plan that you will be likely to follow, it is also important to follow the guidelines for what constitutes an effective program. Most importantly, I urge you to combine both aerobic and anaerobic activities in your exercise program in order to maximize the positive impact for your health, your quality of life, and your weight loss journey.

The Psychology behind the Lifestyle

So far in this book, we've explored many different facets of health, human physiology, calories, nutrition, fitness, exercise, and weight loss. Except for a few brief discussions of the psychological and emotional aspects of obesity, we have focused primarily on the scientific processes that are behind weight gain, exercise, food consumption and digestion, and weight loss.

In a lot of the popular literature about weight loss, dieting, and fitness, I think that there is too much mysticism and fuzzy thinking that is presented to the American public about the reasons *why* so many of us are struggling with overweight and obesity. Many of these same books and weight-loss programs tend to treat the journey towards better health and fitness as some sort of mysterious spiritual quest that can only be completed when you have addressed and resolved all of your emotional issues about overeating, obesity, and life in general.

My own perspective on the issue is far removed from this, and frankly, this tendency in diet and fitness literature makes me angry. I consider it an insult to the intelligence of American adults to focus so exclusively on the emotional, psychological, and spiritual components of obesity and weight loss.

Not that these elements do not form an important function of both the problems and the solutions to the obesity epidemic, on the contrary, these factors *must* be a key component of your journey to fitness. But, at the same time, I think it is more helpful to focus primarily on the physical processes and mechanisms that trigger weight loss, because these are often more tangible and are easier to manipulate than elusive psychological, emotional, and spiritual factors.

This explains why I have spent much of our time together to this point exploring the scientific, medical, and physical aspects of obesity and weight loss. To bend a quote of Thomas Edison's in order to suit my own purposes here, the process of weight loss is 99% perspiration and 1% inspiration.

In other words, if you put in the effort in terms of physical exertion and mindful, careful food consumption, you *will* lose weight. However, at the same time, you have to recognize that without making the mental effort of committing your time and dedication to the journey toward fitness and improved health, you will be unlikely to succeed in this endeavor.[41]

A big part of my problem with the multi-billion dollar diet industry today is that it is populated by many sages, spokespeople, and gurus who do not seem to be that involved in the lifestyle that they are selling you, the consumer. Not to name any names, but it seems pretty obvious that a lot of the major figures in the diet industry do not have the degree of discipline and commitment to fitness and moderation that they are preaching about in their books and television programs, and this kind of hypocrisy really angers me.

My desire to help you on your weight loss journey is born out of the opposite impulse—I would never ask you to do anything that I do not do each and every day of my own life as part of my deep commitment to spreading the news about the benefits of a healthy lifestyle. The plain truth is that part of that commitment means making the personal decision to make strong food choices and maintain my physical fitness on a daily basis.

In other words, the key to improving your health, losing weight, and increasing your physical fitness lies not only in the work of exercising and eating right, but also in renewing your commitment to the process every day. Only by doing this will you be able to sustain your journey in the long-term.

I know, I know, I know—I bet you're shaking your head right now and saying that maintaining that kind of commitment on an ongoing basis is probably a lot harder than it sounds. And that, my friends, is why you and I are going to explore the art and science of motivation together in this chapter.

In the previous chapters, we have explored a wide array of scientific findings about fitness, food consumption, obesity, and why our human bodies require such diligence to avoid gaining excess weight. All of this information has been developed and clarified through scientific studies that have been conducted over the course of the last several decades.

Friends, I have good news and bad news. Bad news first: your weight loss journey *simply cannot succeed* if you are not motivated enough to support it in the long-term. The good news is that during the same decades that evolutionary biologists, epidemiologists, and exercise physiologists were making amazing advances in understanding more about the causes and processes that contribute to human fitness and obesity, psychologists have made similar breakthroughs in observing, analyzing, and understanding the complexities of human motivation.

So, you may be asking, "What does this have to do with me and my journey toward better health and fitness?" It means that what once was mysterious about human motivation has now, to a large extent, been studied and broken down into understandable parts that you can use to fuel your own motivation.

This is not to suggest that a single, unified theory of what constitutes the best method for motivating a long-term fitness regimen has been developed. Instead, what has emerged from the scientific literature over the course of the last several decades is a broad spectrum of theories and models that describe the factors and variables that motivate many different kinds of people in many different types of situations and circumstances.

The different attitudes, opinions, personalities, experiences, and belief systems of the people that you encounter on any given day confirms the infinite variety of the individuals that comprise the human race. It is my opinion that even though we all have similarities that link us together, each person's outlook and life history creates a unique individual, much in the same way that scientists say no two snowflakes are the same.

As such, I think it would be underestimating the endless variety and diversity of humanity to assume that everyone could benefit from applying the same approach to motivation in their quest for a healthier lifestyle the way that many of the popular fitness "gurus" do in their books, DVDs, and television programs. Furthermore, if I outlined a single approach to motivation and expected every reader to follow it, it would be highly likely that it would not be applicable to a lot of people's personalities or life circumstances.

Instead, I want to offer you a broad range of motivational theories, methods, and components to support you in your quest for better health, weight loss, and physical fitness. In the span of just a few short decades, a wide array of motivational literature has been published in the leading scholarly journals. Taken together, these advances in research have significantly advanced the collective understanding of what makes humans tick in terms of meeting goals, both in life in general, and specifically relating to fitness, exercise, diet, and weight loss.

My goal in this chapter is to take you through a tour of some of the most important components of motivation that have been developed by scientists and researchers in recent years. For each model or element, I am going to translate the key research findings into plain English and offer a few real-world examples of the ways that you could apply the findings in your fitness regimen on a daily basis.

This will give you the information that you will need to select an approach to ongoing motivation that you think will be the best fit with your lifestyle, personality, and situation. As much as I would like to get to know each reader personally, I think that you are in a much better position than I am to evaluate the choices that will be offered in this chapter and select the most fitting motivational techniques and methods to guide you on your fitness journey.

After we have taken a spin through some of the major pillars of modern motivational theory, I will focus on giving you some practical guidelines and tips for applying whichever motivational technique that you decide on in a consistent and effective manner.

Motivation: The Mental Motor of the Weight Loss Process

Even if you are an avowed exercise-hater, the process of developing a fitness plan is pretty easy. It is the ongoing commitment of dragging yourself out of bed in the morning or forcing yourself to the gym every day after work that requires the real effort.[42]

So what is the difference between the person who gives up on a weight loss plan or fitness regimen after a few days and the person who begins a new exercise schedule and sticks to it for years? This is a question that you have probably puzzled over in the past, maybe as you waved to the parade of joggers and walkers that stream through the neighborhood every morning or evening.

Many of the men and women that I have encountered who are struggling with a weight problem tend to frame this question in terms of their own perceived weakness and failure. However, this type of thinking is more the result of the low self-esteem and lack of self-confidence that is often associated with long-term weight struggles than a clear view of the complex reality of psychological motivation.[43]

Over the last several decades, scientists and psychologists have explored deeply the question of what motivates human beings. If you look at the statistics about weight loss and fitness, it is clear that a lot of people who are desperately unhappy with their fitness level are not succeeding in their desire to develop and sustain a long-term diet and fitness plan.

However, at the same time, if you look at the individual stories and experiences of the people who have succeeded in their journey toward fitness, improved health, and weight loss, you will notice a common theme emerging: virtually all of these people have thought about motivation in a very specific way and used formal techniques to maintain their motivation on a daily basis.

A cynic might conclude that this means only a few people actually have the willpower to succeed at the challenge of achieving and maintaining permanent weight loss. But I prefer to interpret this disparity as indicating that only a relatively small number of people have been successful in the pursuit of identifying and applying the right motivational strategy to support their weight loss efforts.

One of my longstanding criticisms of the multi-billion dollar diet industry is that its leaders all too often focus on gimmicks and tricks that are highly unlikely to work in the long-term, while overlooking the most basic elements of motivational theory, which could actually provide thousands of people who are struggling with the tools that they need to achieve and sustain their weight-loss objectives.

Using the Scientific Research to Find a Motivation Method that Works for You

Over the last several decades, scientists have begun to undertake increasingly sophisticated observations and analyses of the way that motivation functions in the process of developing and adhering to healthy fitness and diet regimens.[44] From both the successes and failures that researchers have observed during this period, we now have access to a wealth of reliable information about what different motivational techniques people call on during the process of losing weight, increasing their fitness level, and improving their health and quality of life.[45]

As I stated before, the result of this research has been a broad spectrum of motivational models and theories that cover virtually every imaginable variable in terms of personality, health problems, fitness challenges, and life circumstances.[46] Some people may believe that the very variety and diversity of motivational models tends to disprove the credibility of them all. I see it as a realistic reflection of the nearly endless diversity of humanity. When it comes to motivation, one size does *not* fit all. It is up to you to assess the information, select an approach that fits you, and apply it diligently and consistently.

You may be asking, why do I have to bother with this formal motivation mumbo-jumbo? Why can't I just get started with my fitness program without thinking about all the psychological stuff? Well, according to recent research that studied the motivational methods used by those beginning a new exercise regimen, only 19% of those who undertake a new fitness plan with no specific motivational model were found to be continuing to adhere to the plan six months later. In contrast, of the participants in the study who had identified and adhered to a specific motivational plan, over *97%* were still exercising on a regular basis six months later.[47]

Selecting a Motivational Plan

Over the last several decades, many of us have accumulated a lot of guilt, fear, and anxiety about the success and consistency of our exercise schedules and weight loss efforts. This may account for the unrealistic, overly ambitious exercise plans that we devise when we decide to make changes in our lives.

It also may account for the ruthless approach that many novice exercisers take to motivating themselves. However, in reality, the "do or die" mentality that figures heavily in the unfocused motivational models that are used by many novice exercisers is often insufficient to support a long-term life-change effort. Study after study has proven that the best approach to motivating yourself is not following the generic plan that someone else has devised, but rather, choosing an approach that is personalized to your criteria, circumstances, personality, and lifestyle.[48]

That is why I think that a crucial ingredient for weight loss success is taking the time to understand the differences and similarities in the leading models of motivation. This process also involves taking stock of your own personality, strengths, and weaknesses, and making an honest, informed determination of what approach to motivation will be the most likely to help you sustain your regimen over time.

What do YOU want to Achieve with Your Fitness Plan?

If your initial reaction was "Duh! Weight loss!" when you read that question, I don't blame you. This is the automatic answer, and it is the one that the propaganda of the multi-billion dollar weight loss industry has emblazoned in all of our minds. But what I want to convey to you with this question is the importance of thinking deeply about what fitness means to you. In truth, weight loss—the physical transformation of the body—is often secondary to our *real* fitness and health-related goals and desires.

For every person, the ultimate objective of the journey to better health, increased fitness, and weight loss is different. But many times, I have found that specific aspects of life quality are a better motivating factor than the vague, generic description of "losing weight." Do you want to be able to feel healthier and more energetic? Socialize without self-consciousness? Actively participate in vigorous activities? Play with your children or grandchildren? Prolong your life? Enjoy your life more? Look better in your clothes?

Once you have identified a few principal reasons for initiating your weight loss journey, take a few minutes to fully consider the wide ripple of implications and consequences that these changes will have in your every day life. For example, instead of generalities like "participating in more vigorous activities," "socializing with self-confidence," or "looking better in my clothes," begin to allow yourself to think in more specific terms of the way that improved fitness will resonate within your daily life.

Particularize your goals. Think about joining a club or an organization that you have always been interested in. Think about taking up tennis, or rock-climbing, or square-dancing, or some other activity that you have not been able to bring yourself to contemplate while you are out of shape. Think about your new shape in that special outfit that you have saved at the back of your closet.

What I am trying to illustrate here is that a vital part of developing an effective approach to motivation is considering what about improving your health and losing weight means to you. Not what it *should* mean to you, according to the views perpetuated by the gurus and prophets of the multi-billion diet industry. Rather, you must determine what the large and small changes in your health, fitness, and body *will* mean to you on a daily basis.

Doing some serious thinking about what objectives you are seeking to achieve with your lifestyle changes is the first step to devising a meaningful, effective approach to motivation that will sustain you throughout the process of your health and fitness journey. This is the kernel of scientific fact that underlies the sentiment that has now become a weight-loss cliché: "It will only work if you are doing it for yourself." My only modification of this motto would be that weight loss only works if you have clearly identified your objectives and you renew your commitment to these goals on a daily basis.

The Components of Fitness Motivation

There have been literally thousands of scholarly studies and academic journal articles that have explored various aspects of exercise motivation over the last several decades. I have looked over a lot of them, both in the process of devising a rational, scientifically-based plan for my own fitness regimen and in researching this book.

There are more theories and models about motivation than I could ever list in the confines of a single chapter, and many of them are so specific and targeted that they cannot really be applied in everyday situations by a wide variety of people. However, through the process of extensively searching the literature on these subjects, I noticed that a number of themes and ideas were consistently repeated, even when the researchers who were reporting on the results of different studies were using slightly divergent phrases and terminology to refer to these concepts.

Drawing on these similarities, I am going to discuss a number of the components of an effective motivational plan. However, the task of determining which of these factors is more important to you and which will, therefore, serve as the centerpiece of your personalized approach to motivation, is up to you.

The Buddy System: Social Support and Involvement

One element that is mentioned again and again in the fitness motivation research is the importance, to some people, of placing your fitness, health improvement, and weight-loss goals into a social context. For many complex reasons that have to do with our degree of social orientation, many people are more apt to feel obligated to stick to a new fitness and diet regimen if that vow has been made publicly.[49]

Indeed, some of the most effective fitness and weight-loss programs have been based upon this concept. A number of recent studies have manipulated the participants' sense of social obligation as a means of ensuring their continuing commitment to an exercise plan.

Some researchers have taken this idea to the extreme by devising a fitness plan that involves the formation of small teams that are comprised of co-workers, neighbors, friends, or family members, although some degree of formality and social distance is necessary to maximize the benefits of a sense of social obligation.

Then, each team member contributes a monetary contribution. If *any* of the team members fails to adhere to the exercise plan that they developed for themselves, *all* of the team members lose their money. Although this arrangement is somewhat unorthodox, it has proven to be very effective by exploiting the unwillingness to let others down and the avoidance of public humiliation that are both longstanding traits of human society. This is an extreme form of using social ties as a way of maintaining your motivation to adhere to your fitness and weight-loss plan.

There are other methods that are based on the same principle, all of which share an element of heightened accountability.[50] Some people create groups or duos who commit to exercise together on a regular schedule. Others start personal logs on the Internet that they use to report their daily activities and progress to an audience of both friends and strangers. The national weight-loss programs that use a weekly group weigh-in as a cornerstone of their system are also operating on the same principle of accountability.

Others turn to social support as a means of easing what they regard as the drudgery of exercising.[51] By committing to an evening walk with a friend or neighbor, the unpleasantness that you may have long associated with physical exertion could be exchanged for the pleasure of social interaction. Several studies have confirmed that exercising or engaging on a weight-loss plan with a partner or a group exponentially increases one's chances of success.[52]

However, the social element is likely to vary in importance according to your personality. If you are an introvert who shies away from social interaction, exercising with a buddy may be akin to submitting to physical torture. Likewise, if you have a propensity to renege on promises with no regrets or remorse, an accountability-based weight-loss program is unlikely to be particularly effective for you. Once again, assessing your own situation before you choose an approach to motivation is of central importance to guaranteeing your success.

Creating a Realistic Balance between Fitness and Your Life

There is an important equilibrium that you must achieve when you are seeking to initiate a program that will help you lose weight, increase your fitness level, and improve your health and quality of life. When you are developing a personalized system, you have to make sure that you are going to change your lifestyle enough to result in significant, tangible changes in your overall fitness and weight.[53] However, at the same time, you do not want to devise a plan that necessitates that you must engage in behaviors and activities that bear no resemblance whatsoever to your real life.

Part of the propaganda that has emerged from the multi-billion dollar diet industry has been an idealized vision of fitness. In infomercials and public service announcements, we have been exposed to visions of an alternate universe when every man, woman, and child has hours each day to devote solely to fitness and weight loss.

You and I both know that this simply is not the case. Throughout this book, I have tried to impress upon you that I recognize that modern life is often so hectic, rushed, and chock-full of responsibilities that finding time to devote to positive lifestyle changes often seems impossible. A major weakness of many beginners' fitness and weight loss plans is that they devise ambitious regimens that, if followed, would devour almost all of their free time. I have always viewed this type of beginner's ambition as understandable and admirable but highly likely to result in inconsistency, disappointment, and ultimately failure.

The research on the subject backs up my impression of the dangers of succumbing to this kind of over-ambitious planning.[54] It turns out that one of the most significant factors in determining whether people adhere to a weight loss program is the degree of ease and convenience with which the exercise and diet plan can be reconciled to other life responsibilities.[55] Not surprisingly, a number of studies have proven that fitness and weight loss plans that are highly convenient are those that participants adhere to most consistently.

As I have encountered men and women who are struggling with obesity, a common complaint that I have heard is that many people feel that their busy schedules do not allow sufficient time for the aerobics, anaerobic exercise, and healthy food preparation that weight loss and fitness requires. As someone who runs a company that requires my full-time commitment, I understand the juggling of responsibilities that often has to be done in order to fit these activities in.

The first step of solving any problem in life is assessment. As I recommended in the discussion of defining your own personal weight loss goals and motivations, the first part of the process of finding the time that is necessary to devote to fitness and healthy eating is taking a hard, honest look at the way that you spend your time on a typical day. Instead of estimating your daily schedule and the time that must be dedicated to each responsibility, set aside a week during which you religiously record every activity and how much time you devoted to it.

Many times, people invest more hours than they realize to low-value activities like television. If you are unwilling to give up or reduce your nightly TV time, maybe the best solution is purchasing equipment that you can use to exercise while watching television, such as a treadmill or a stair climbing machine, both of which can be gotten for relatively low prices these days.

If these are out of your price range, or if you prefer a low-tech approach, options such as mini-trampolines, skipping rope, or jogging in place are all possibilities that could be combined with your nightly television time. This brainstorming process can be applied to your entire schedule in order to shave off wasted minutes, multi-task, or identify openings that you could finesse in time for exercising.

The key is achieving a balance between changing your life enough that you will not easily fall back into bad habits, but not so much that the changes will be unsustainable in the long-term.[56] The research on the subject proves conclusively that too much inconvenience is a factor that will inevitably kill the motivation that you need to make a positive, lasting change in your health, fitness, and weight.[57]

Believing in Your Ability to Change: Understanding Self-Efficacy

You may not be familiar with the concept that behavioral psychologists refer to as "self-efficacy," but it is a vital component of motivation.[58] Although self-efficacy is a complex concept, it can basically be explained as the degree of confidence that you have in your ability to follow through with the goals that you have set for yourself.

The factors that influence our degree of self-efficacy are multi-faceted. However, having a history of failed or abandoned attempts at weight loss can contribute to a low level of confidence in your ability to succeed in future attempts. Even if your belief in your ability to achieve your goals is overly optimistic or irrational, scientists have observed, you are far more likely to succeed than a person who does not possess a high degree of self-efficacy.[59]

The good news is that the research also shows that self-efficacy can be deliberately cultivated over time, particularly with regard to fitness and weight loss regimens. Experts recommend setting smaller, interim goals and measures of performance, rather than focusing on the entirety of your targeted weight loss at once.[60]

If you chart your progress and exercise on a daily basis, you are more likely to develop a sense of moving forward in the process of weight loss, as well as to gain a sense of optimism and confidence in your ability to stick to a plan. Over time, the sense of achievement that you accumulate from these small victories will result in significant gains in your overarching sense of self-efficacy. In this way, the benefits that you gain from looking at your fitness goals and achievements in a more positive, productive manner can increase your chances of long-term success exponentially.

Intrinsic vs. Extrinsic Motivation

Another important component of understanding and using the most effective approach to motivation to support your physical fitness program can be found in differentiating between intrinsic and extrinsic motivation.[61] This is a concept that has been part of the psychological literature for years, but in recent studies, it has emerged as an important factor in weight loss and fitness research.[62]

Extrinsic motivation is defined as a motivating factor that is external and outcome-oriented, such as studying to get good grades or working for a paycheck.[63] In contrast, intrinsic motivation is the process of being motivated by the process and the inherent value of the activity, rather than its expected outcome. For example, most people pursue their hobbies and leisure activities based on intrinsic motivation.

Extrinsic motivation can be a compelling reason to achieve success in the short-term. However, the vast majority of the research on the subject suggests that goals that are intrinsically motivated are more likely to be achieved and sustained, because they have a deeper, more personal meaning for the individual pursuing them.[64]

There are a number of techniques that you can use to increase your intrinsic motivation for fitness and weight loss. First, it may help to focus more on the benefits of the *process* of becoming fit, rather than the ultimate outcome. For example, many people experience increased energy and heightened moods after exercising. These could function as intrinsic motivation to continue with your daily fitness routine.

Furthermore, experts note that it is important to consciously link your fitness activities to your larger value system in order to increase your intrinsic motivation. For example, if you see your daily exercise as expressing gratitude for your health, or if you conceptualize your healthy eating habits as part of your stewardship of your body, this could heighten intrinsic motivation, which, in turn, is associated with long-term success in the weight loss literature.

Tying It All Together: Sustaining the Challenge of Motivation

In this chapter, I've outlined some of the basic components of motivation that have been developed in research literature in recent years. The exact approach that will work for you can only be determined by you, after you have taken an honest survey of your personality, strengths, weaknesses, and past efforts. The more you have carefully considered your own motivational needs, the more fitting a plan you will be able to devise and the greater your chances of long-term success.[65]

The only constant that must be a non-negotiable part of every person's motivation plan is making the daily, ongoing effort to diligently and carefully maintain your commitment to fitness, weight loss, and improved health. It is a daily struggle, and all too often, our hectic lives seem to be conspiring against our commitment to positive change. But in the end, the responsibility to renew your commitment and dedication to your goals is yours, and yours alone.

Action: Beyond Setting Goals

Journaling: The Key to Lasting Health and Fitness

Creating Awareness of Your Habits

As I have stated several times in this book, I am decidedly *not* one of those weight loss "experts" who does not seem to understand the pressures, responsibilities, and hectic schedules that are involved in the daily lives of the people who are facing weight loss challenges and fitness issues. To read some of the fitness plans that are out there, you would think that nobody had to work or take care of outside responsibilities and that people had infinite amounts of free time dedicated to careful meal planning—meticulously weighing of food portions and ingredients—and intricately complicated fitness programs.

Like you, I have a "day job" outside of the fitness industry, as well as a family with the hundreds of big and little responsibilities that family life entails on a daily basis. On a profound level, I understand the intense pressure and responsibilities that "normal" people face on a daily basis because I have the same type of challenges, responsibilities, and obligations. The only difference that separates me from millions of other working men and women is that I have made a personal commitment to fitness. As such, I regard my daily workouts and healthy eating plan to be a non-negotiable component of my life, as important and unavoidable as brushing my teeth or going to work.

Modern life is busy, often to the point of insanity. But being busy does not necessarily prevent you from being healthy, and I am walking proof of that. The pitfall that many people have stumbled into is eating quickly (and often poorly) on the run, failing to exercise consistently, and never giving a lot of thought to either one of these important aspects of health. Truth be told, you would probably be able to function a lot more effectively in fulfilling the responsibilities of your busy lifestyle if you put just a little more effort into making sure that you were eating right and working out on a regular basis.

Unfortunately, a lot of people get caught up in the thought process that sees eating as just another item on a seemingly endless to-do list. As a result, many tend to eat as quickly as possible, sometimes only semi-conscious of the quantity, quality, characteristics, and health impact of what is being put into their bodies as fuel for their busy lives.

The first step to making major, lasting changes to your health and fitness is regaining an awareness of exactly what you are eating, doing, thinking, and feeling throughout the course of the day. In reality, the only effective way to increase your consciousness of the food you consume and the time you spend engaged in unproductive, low-value activities is to create a journal. I have often heard it said that the path to any journey starts with a first step. However, if that first step is taken without preparing for the journey, you may be wandering around forever. If you were going to travel from California to New York, you would probably invest in a good map before you began your journey. A fitness journal is just like a good map. If you want to lose weight or get into better shape, you have to figure out how to get there. You must know the path before you take that first step.

Each one of us is a unique individual, with different motivations, experiences, and reactions. As such, our journals will likely take vastly different directions and forms, and that's okay—I want your journal to be a place where you can reflect, analyze, plan, and envision whatever seems most crucial to your own mental and physical well-being.

However, that being said, there are also a number of key components that *must* be present in your journal in order to ensure that it will be effective. These components include food intake, physical activity, and personal thoughts and reflections.

Journaling your eating patterns and daily food intake involves transcribing all of the food and beverages that you eat and drink every day. This is pretty self-explanatory, but ensuring accuracy and detail are key issues to the degree of effectiveness that you will get out of this activity.

It is also important to write down the exercise and physical activity that you do every day. This should be limited to the preplanned activities that you engage in on a daily basis. For example, my own preplanned exercise routine includes both aerobic and anaerobic components, and I note these in my daily journal as soon as I have completed them, both as a means of documenting my physical activity and motivating my future performance.

If you happen to engage in some unplanned physical activity, such as helping a friend move to a new house or walking the mall, it is not necessary to note this in your journal, because it's not a core part of your planned fitness routine. Although you will probably get some physical benefit from these types of activities, they don't count as exercise in the important formal sense.

The third component of the journal is equally important, but the exact form and shape that it takes is up to you. In whatever manner feels meaningful and helpful, you should record your daily thoughts, feelings, reactions, challenges, inspirations, and motivations. These can be positive or negative—the important thing is being honest with yourself in the process.

I like to use my journal to document and then analyze my feelings. In other words, if I found that I had a negative or pessimistic reaction to a new challenge in my workout routine, I record it, try to identify the origins of this reaction, and then I try to reshape it through visualization and positive thinking. It is not enough to simply dump out your feelings; I want you to use your journal to proactively assess and direct these feelings in a productive way.

I can practically hear you moaning in exasperation right now! Don't worry; I am not going to try to force you to tote around a three-ring binder and make detailed, *War and Peace*-length notes about your daily food intake, exercise, and other items. But in order to gain true awareness about what you are putting into your body, it is crucial that you take the steps to make sure that you are prepared to jot down basic facts about the time, amount, and types of food and beverages that you are consuming.

Just as an example, try to remember what you ate last Tuesday. Can you come up with a detailed account of your food intake and exercise, or your feelings that day? I am willing to bet the answer is probably a resounding "No."

However, because I have made journaling a non-negotiable part of my daily routine for several decades, I can flip back to any given day over the past twenty years and recount these facts. I am convinced that having this record of my progress has been a key part of my continued success on my own journey towards better health and fitness.

I encourage people to keep a fitness journal throughout the weight loss process, but it is particularly important during the first week or so of the program. In fact, before you are even considering diving into a weight loss program full-force, it may be beneficial to start a fitness journal.

For a lot of men and women, seeing what types and amounts of food that they are actually eating on a daily basis can be a real eye-opener. Often, we have an idealized notion of our diet that does not actually match our actions. Keeping a food diary will put you on the path to awareness, and awareness is vital in order to help you make strong, healthy food choices as you begin to lose weight and journey towards improved health and fitness.

While journaling will help you to gain awareness and control over the amount of calories that you are consuming, it will have an even greater impact in the area of exercise. What may seem like a pointless exercise in futility is probably a slow but definite course of improvement, and journals can prove it.

For example, when I first started my aerobic activity, I was huffing and puffing to last 5 minutes on a stationary bike, set at the lowest level; the next day I would try for 6 minutes, than 7 minutes, and so on. Within 2 months, I was riding for 30 minutes at maximum intensity. Now, it may take you a little longer to achieve maximum intensity, but the main idea is that with a journal, you can see your gradual improvement over time and take comfort in even small incremental achievements in your progress.

Like I said, I am not recommending an overly detailed journal; however, the greater the detail, the greater the probability for long term success. To start with, just keep a small notebook or scrap of paper handy to note the times, amounts, and types of foods and drinks that you consume every day. Remember, no cheating! This process won't help you gain awareness if you are not fully truthful in your journal. And contrary to popular belief, the scraps you pick off of your kids' plates while filling the dishwasher *do* contain calories.

Another tool that has been introduced recently seems to be enormously helpful to people who are trying to keep track of their food intake is online food tracking. There are a number of different online food journals that are available. With just a few clicks of the mouse, these tools can help you keep a detailed, accurate account of what you have eaten every day. They can also track nutrients such as calories, vitamins, fat, and other variables.

Now, there are several pay sites that will charge you to keep an online food journal—steer clear of these. They are often affiliated with expensive, ineffective proprietary weight loss programs. Instead, it is better to pick one of the free sites that provide online food journaling capabilities.

There are many such sites available on the Internet today, though they may advertise products for sale, it is not necessary to buy anything. I have heard of other people who have started free "web logs"—blogs, for short—to help them keep track of their food intake and stay accountable. No matter which approach you prefer, journaling is a vital part of the weight loss process and fitness plan.

Food: Let's Eat

Calories In, Calories Out

Let's talk six-packs. And no, I'm not referring to your favorite beverage. I'm talking about that ever-elusive set of muscles called the abdominals. Abs, Abs, Abs. People spend hundreds of thousands of dollars every year on a quest to develop and refine this widely-admired body part. Whether the owner of said six-pack is male or female, admirers seem to be universally mystified when they spot a well-chiseled set of abdominals framed by a fit body.

The unique and persistent allure of the abdominal muscles can be traced back to the aesthetic sensibility of the ancient Greeks, who created the first gymnasiums. Greek culture placed a high premium on athletic ability stressing diet and exercising rather than drugs for maintaining health. And for better or for worse, their culture also tended to equate beauty with virtue. Taken together, these two elements resulted in an appreciation for an eye-pleasing midriff that has persisted long past the expiration date of other ancient Greek practices, such as a penchant for toga fashions and naked wrestling.

Since the time of Socrates, who kept himself in great physical condition, contemporary societies have remained infatuated with well-toned abdominal muscles, even as other trends and fads about body shapes and ideal beauty have come and gone throughout history. As a result, people have developed many techniques and methods intended to sculpt and shape these appealing muscles, many of which have been ill-advised and even downright dangerous.

If I had a nickel for every time I have been asked "How do you get Abs like yours?" over the past twenty years, I'd have long since settled into the most luxurious villa on Easy Street. The questions I get are often fraught with confusion and desperation: Do I need to do thousands of sit-ups? Have you tried the Six Minute Ab Machine? Body by Jake? The Ab Roller? Inverted crunches? Bends? Lunges? Twists? Dips? Liposuction? Voodoo?

Unfortunately, the secret of well-defined Abs is not to be found in an infomercial (or voodoo rituals). What all of these questions and queries reveal is a misunderstanding of the role that body fat plays in your muscle definition. You can do crunches until the cows come home, but if your stomach is covered in rolls of fat, nobody will be able to appreciate your efforts. You have to work on diminishing your overall body fat before you can even begin to worry about achieving and honing muscular definition.

Sadly, abdominal fat is often highly resistant to just exercise. Have you ever noticed people who are regularly exercising—bicycle riding, playing tennis, swimming, going to the gym, or other activities—and who presumably eat healthy food—tofu, yogurt, soy milk, and wheat-grass juice—but who are never able to lose the fat around their mid-section? That's more than likely because those people are continuing to take in more calories than they are expending. In other words, they are still overeating. So how do we go about solving this conundrum that has left so many people desperately confused? Well, we need start with the basics: determining your total daily calorie needs.

The first step is determining your *Basal Metabolic Rate* (BMR). This is the amount of energy (measured in calories) that your body needs to take in to support your basic bodily functions and ensure your continuing survival.

In order to calculate your BMR, use the following equation and plug in your personal weight, height, and age data:

FOR ADULT MALES:

66 + (6.3 X body weight in pounds) + (12.9 X height in inches) – (6.8 X age in years) = targeted daily caloric intake

66	+	(6.3 x ___ lbs.)	+	(12.9 x ___ inches tall)	-	(6.8 x ___ age)	=	Basal Metabolic Rate (BMR)
66	+	(_____)	+	(_____)	-	(_____)	=	_____ Basal Metabolic Rate (BMR)

Example:

Male, 30 years old, weighing 250 pounds, 5 feet 10 inches tall

66	+	(6.3 x 250 lbs.)	+	(12.9 x 70 inches tall)	-	(6.8 x 30 age)	=	Basal Metabolic Rate (BMR)
66	+	(1575)	+	(903)	-	(204)	=	2340 Basal Metabolic Rate (BMR)

FOR ADULT FEMALES:

655 + (4.3 X body weight in pounds) + (4.7 X height in inches) – (4.7 X age in years) = targeted daily caloric intake

655	+	(4.3 x ___ lbs.)	+	(4.7 x ___ inches tall)	-	(4.7 x ___ age)	=	Basal Metabolic Rate (BMR)
655	+	(_____)	+	(_____)	-	(_____)	=	_____ Basal Metabolic Rate (BMR)

Example:

Female, 28 years old, weighing 225 pounds, 5 feet 5 inches tall

655	+	(4.3 x 225 lbs.)	+	(4.7 x 65 inches tall)	-	(4.7 x 28 age)	=	Basal Metabolic Rate (BMR)
655	+	(967.5)	+	(305.5)	-	(131.6)	=	1796.4 Basal Metabolic Rate (BMR)

The second step is determining your *Total Daily Calorie Needs.* In order to arrive at this figure, you simply multiply your BMR by the Activity Multiplier that best indicates your activity level.

Activity Multiplier (used for both men and women)

- If you are sedentary (little or no exercise, office job), multiply your basal metabolic rate by 1.2
- If you are slightly active (light exercise/sports 1-3 days per week), multiply your basal metabolic rate by 1.375
- If you are moderately active (moderate exercise/sports 3-5 days per week), multiply your basal metabolic rate by 1.55
- If you engage in heavy exercise (hard exercise/sports 6-7 days per week) multiply your basal metabolic rate by 1.725

Sedentary Female Example

BMR	X	Activity Multiplier	=	Total Daily Calories
1796.4	X	1.2	=	2156 Total Daily Calories (rounded up)

Next, round off the number = 2156 Total Daily Calorie Needs.

Your Total Daily Calories

BMR	X	Activity Multiplier	=	Total Daily Calories
____	X	____	=	____Total Daily Calories (rounded up)

Now that you know your total daily calorie needs, let's see how it relates to meals. Because you should not go more than 3 or 4 hours between eating, you will need to divide your total daily calorie needs into 4-6 meals each day.

Using the example above, you can create a meal plan that is tailored directly to your personal needs. For example, to determine how many calories to eat in four meals, you would divide 2156 calories by 4. This results in four meals of roughly 539 calories each. Dividing by 5 would result in 5 meals of 431 calories each, while dividing by 6 would result 6 meals of 359 calories each.

You can play with these numbers by having a little more at one meal and a little less at another, as your schedule, hunger patterns, and needs change. The key to remember is that you should never consume more calories than two meals at any one time. Remember that it is impossible to fool your body; it will inevitably store any excess unused calories from overeating as fat.

Cheat Meal

When you combine your total daily calorie needs with a formal exercise program, you will be at a calorie deficit. This deficit will eventually lead to a reduction of body fat. However, once a week, you are going to be required to cheat at one meal. That's right: I am ordering you to *cheat* on your diet.

At the end of each week, you choose one meal that will be your cheat meal. At that meal, you are allowed to eat whatever, and as much, as you want. If you want to eat nothing but cake and ice cream, go ahead, have as much of it as your heart desires. Your choice may not be to eat junk food, but you should eat as much of whatever you choose at one sitting.

The cheat meal serves two purposes:

1. It is a reward for working hard all week long, and it will be something to look forward to every week.
2. More importantly, it will allow your metabolism to fluctuate and your energy to increase.

Once you have reached your fitness goal, your cheat meal can be expanded to a cheat day. But remember: Do not cheat more than one meal each week until you have reached your fitness goal!

Food

If you have any experience reading diet and fitness books, you have probably noticed a big difference between this book and some of the other books you have read before: I have not mentioned what you can and can't eat. That's because I believe that you should eat a wide assortment of foods, and that no foods should be forbidden.

I believe that this approach is a crucial part of maintaining health goals, as well as helping you to avoid binge eating. Excluding foods that are enjoyable can lead an individual to overindulge during times of frailty, stress, or anxiety. It is far more important to understand which foods contribute to your calorie intake.

In general, foods that contain the largest number of calories per volume or weight are those that are higher in fat. A calorie is a calorie for the purpose of controlling weight; 100 calories of white meat chicken is the same as 100 calories of chocolate cake. However, when you start taking particular note of the relative calorie densities of different foods in combination with a formal exercise program, you will start to adjust your food choices for more satisfying and healthy options.

Nutritional needs can differ according to the lifestyle of each individual. One so-called expert, in a recent bestselling book on fitness, listed meals that would comprise a "Perfect Eating Day." I feel that this sort of absolutism is utterly ridiculous. What works for one person may not work for another. For example, because I choose to train with weights in order to sculpt my body, my nutritional needs incorporate a higher percentage of protein, fewer carbohydrates and only minimal fats. However, a person who has more of an aerobic lifestyle, such as a bicycle racer, would need to consume more carbohydrates and less protein, while a boxer preparing for a fifteen-round bout may need more fats than carbohydrates in order to sustain the grueling punishment that the body will encounter. I believe that the perfect eating day is what works for *you* and not what someone else believes you should eat.

I would suggest that you start by assuming that 40 percent of your total daily calories should come from quality proteins found in chicken, fish, turkey, lean meats, or egg whites; with 40 percent coming from carbohydrates (this would include vegetables and fruits, as well as whole grain breads, pasta, rice, and potatoes). Fats can account for the last 20 percent of your caloric intake.

The following is an example of one of my own morning meals: eight egg whites and two egg yolks; 4 ounces of white meat chicken with mushrooms; and 1 whole grain English muffin (no butter). This meal is approximately 570 calories. For a more aerobic lifestyle, I might replace the chicken with the same calorie amount of potatoes.

While the majority of my meals cater to my lifestyle and my weight-lifting-influenced diet, I have also been known to stop at a Starbucks on my way home from the gym in the morning for coffee and a piece of lemon loaf cake. However, I make sure that I count this splurge in my total daily calorie needs. Remember, it's all about balancing and enjoying your life.

Exercising: Pursuing a Fit Lifestyle

Straight from the Heart

The decision to incorporate an exercise program into your life is not one that should be taken lightly. In order to fully reap the benefits of your time and effort, your investment and commitment to fitness must be lifelong. Just as brushing your teeth is a non-negotiable part of daily life, you have to commit to exercise consistently, without questions or excuses. You must be absolutely convinced that the benefits of exercise far outweigh the risk of a sedentary lifestyle.

True fitness success can only be achieved by those who understand that excellence is not something that you can go out and buy, but rather, can only be found in the courage to fight against the odds. I have a profound respect for the men and women who have chosen to adopt a fit lifestyle and pursue that goal with tenacity, dedication, consistency, and commitment.

In my own experience, I have witnessed many people who appeared to visit the gym in order to work on their social muscles: "talking the talk." They're the same ones who wonder why they never seem to get into shape even though they go to the gym 5 or 6 days a week. Now, I'm not saying you shouldn't be friendly or avoid saying hello to those you meet in the gym, but avoid long conversations or ongoing commitments, because you are there to *work*. Don't get me wrong; one of the things that I love about working out is the friendly energy and hustle-and-bustle of the gym. However, if you ask anyone who has seen me exercising, they'll tell you that I train hard and I don't screw around.

I have chosen not to candy-coat this section the way that other so-called experts have. They may want you to think that building a fit physique is easy, but the truth is that it simply isn't. Hard work and patience are essential. I did not develop my body by using a ThighMaster or the latest Bowflex home gym. I didn't get this way in 12 short weeks using the Skinny Life Diet. While most people were still sleeping, I was up early, at the gym, transforming myself physically, mentally, and even spiritually. You cannot hope to erase in a few days or weeks what a lifetime of sedentary living has bestowed. But you *can* get there in time; just don't give up.

How often, how fast, and how long you exercise is up to you. These determinations should be made based on the fitness goals that you have set for yourself. If you're male or female, young or old, a beginner or advanced, overweight or underweight, the intensity must be the same in relative terms. What I mean is that whether you are lifting 3 pounds or 300 hundred pounds, at the lowest level on the aerobic scale or the highest level, you should be giving the maximum effort for your ability. Follow me on this journey and I can promise you physical fitness and the well-being that it entails. Remember, when you finally push yourself beyond anything you ever thought was physically possible for you to do, I have been there too, and I will continue walking the walk towards lifelong fitness alongside you.

Pre-Workout

Know what you are going to do before you do it.

First of all, you have to decide how many days a week you are going to devote to your exercise program. Then you must know every step of your routine before you start in order to maximize your time investment.

I cannot tell you how many times I've seen people walk into the gym with no idea of what they are going to do. They'll spend 10 minutes just trying to figure out what to do, and then flounder around without accomplishing much of anything. Adhering to a predetermined schedule will provide the structure that you need to ensure that your time spent exercising will be effective and efficient.

I will offer a number of sample workout schedules. You can always rearrange the days and exercises to accommodate your schedule. If you like them, use them. If not, switch them around, depending on your schedule, availability, goals, and physical needs. Try not to be lazy about it, though; what you put into your fitness regimen is what you'll get out of it. I currently train 6 days a week, using a 4-day split routine. In addition, I do 20 minutes of aerobic activity every day.

Day #1—Chest
Day #2—Back and Biceps
Day #3—Shoulders and Triceps
Day #4—Legs, including calves
Day #5—Repeat day #1
Day #6—Repeat day #2

I usually take Sunday off and pick up on Monday where I left off on Saturday; in this way, each muscle group gets worked three times during a two week period. I choose not to work my abdominals much, but you could work yours each day if you'd like. Remember, though, you will not be able to see definition in your abs unless you have established a sufficient calorie deficit to remove the fat that is most likely covering them.

A *5-day routine* might look like this:

Monday—Chest
Tuesday—Back
Wednesday—Shoulders

Thursday—Arms (Biceps and Triceps)
Friday—Legs

This routine would work well for those that want the weekend off.

A routine incorporating 3 days per week is the minimum requirement to maintain your current fitness level; I would not recommend this unless you absolutely cannot find additional time in your schedule to train.

A *3-day routine* might look like this:

Monday—Chest and Back
Wednesday—Shoulders and Arms
Friday—Legs

If you decide on a 3-day workout schedule, you must make sure that you continually put out maximum effort during your training. You will need to put more pressure on the muscles throughout every workout in order to see effective results.

The routines that you need to build muscle definition are simple to perform. Sets and reps are the building blocks of your routine. A rep (repetition) is one complete execution of an exercise. So, for example, one rep is one full up-and-down movement of a strength exercise. A set is comprised of reps performed until failure—yes, *failure*, meaning that you cannot prompt your body to perform another rep. A good rule of thumb is to keep your reps between 12 and 15 to condition your muscle or between 6 and 8 to increase muscle size.

You should incorporate a primary exercise and a secondary exercise for larger muscle groups such as chest, back, and legs. Primary exercises develop the health and strength of the muscles, while secondary exercises shape and sculpt the muscle.

The intensity should be the same whether you want to condition or build your muscles; find a weight you can lift for the maximum reps in the first set (any exercise). I would recommend that beginners start with one primary exercise for each muscle group consisting of 2-3 sets for each exercise. You will not be able to do the maximum reps for each set, but keep in mind that this last rep should be a real struggle. Now you train with this weight until you are able to do all 3 sets for the maximum reps. Once you reach this level, start adding a little weight to the exercise (don't worry, ladies, you will not build muscles like a man!).

The Workout

Warming up the Body

Warm up your body before you start your pre-planned exercise routine. The idea is to gradually increase your heart rate, expand tissue elasticity, and prepare yourself mentally for sustained physical exertion. This can be done in a variety of ways; however, according to the American College of Sports Medicine, stretching should not be considered a warm-up movement, as it can lead to injuries of cold muscles. If you want to stretch before working out, make sure you warm up first. Light calisthenics, such as knee lifts, arm circles, or trunk rotations, are good movements for warming up. I have found that low intensity movements that stimulate the muscle movement to be used in the activity work well for me. Also, spending 3-5 minutes on a stationary bike at a low intensity is a great warm-up. For convenience, you could continue on at a higher level for your daily aerobic activity once you have completed a short warm-up.

Aerobic Activity

When I started my fitness journey several decades ago, about the only forms of aerobic activities that were popular at the time were jogging, running, or stationary bicycles that resembled medieval torture machines. Today, there are hundreds of different aerobic activities and equipment that can help you to get your cardiovascular system into top shape. Some are good, and some are not so good, depending on your reasons for using them and your fitness goals.

One basic rule of thumb that I have found to be helpful is to keep it simple and stick to the basics whenever possible. For example, one piece of equipment that I didn't find to be advantageous was a recumbent bike that had a monitor attached to it allowing the users to access the Internet while exercising. This idea might sound good, but the men and women I observed on the machine would often pay too much attention to the Internet and not enough to the work at hand. Try to avoid bells and whistles and other distractions that may keep you from concentrating on your training.

Some of my aerobic favorites are the stationary bikes (now tremendously improved from the old days), elliptical machines, and the treadmills for a fast walk. On sunny days, I enjoy peddling my beach cruiser along Pacific Cost Highway, glancing at the endless parade of waves crashing on the sandy shoreline as I build up a good sweat. I don't like to run because of the continuous pounding on the knees, but if you enjoy running try to stay off hard surfaces and use good shoes. Although I am not a big fan of aerobic classes, they do seem to work well for many people; just don't forget your strength training.

Strength Training

There are thousands of exercise routines that can be performed according to an individual's particular needs; however, there are some fundamental exercises that you must master before even contemplating advanced movements. If you have been working out for some time with little discernible result, you probably did not master the basics.

These basic movements work all the major muscles in the body—chest, back, shoulders, arms, and legs. While changing exercises now and then can be a benefit to your overall program, classic exercises should not be changed because of their time-proven ability to sculpt and expedite muscle development.

It's normal to feel awkward when you initially undertake any activity that you are not familiar with, but it doesn't take long to improve your skills if you stick with it. The saying "practice makes perfect" may be a cliché, but in many ways, it's fundamentally true. Remember, everyone starts out as a beginner. Just work at your own level, start out slow, and gradually increase the duration and level of difficulty as your fitness level and physical development progress.

Demonstrating an assortment of exercises by means of still photos, such as the ones depicted in fitness magazines and books can generate an illusion of the exercise's true movement. I witness people performing fundamental exercises incorrectly every day, even though they've read the books and looked through the magazines. It's difficult to view yourself while performing an exercise, even with the aid of mirrors. Common mistakes include arching the back too much, using legs muscles in order to facilitate an upper body movement, and not incorporating the full range of motion. This is especially important for men to remember, because many men attempt to lift too much weight too rapidly, and in doing so, not only miss the benefits of the exercise, but also significantly increase the chance of injury. A professional fitness trainer or a good training partner can help curtail common mistakes and be an advantage to your overall success.

As an example: this morning I observed a young lady performing an Incline Dumbbell Press; this is an advanced movement, and I do not recommend it for beginners. Although her range of motion was respectable, her hips were off the bench as she pressed with her legs in order to aid in lifting the dumbbells above her chest. This is a frequent error when individuals try to lift too much weight. Remember, as I have said many times before, becoming fit is not an overnight process; it's a lifestyle commitment that will yield results in the long-term.

As an instructor, I monitor the overall movement of the exercise for maximum efficiency. Through the mirror image I make sure that feet are flat on the floor, legs are not used to assist with the lift, hips and upper back stay flat on the bench to minimizing the use of secondary muscles such as the shoulders and triceps. I also lend support on the last few repetitions to fully exhaust the muscle being worked. This allows the lifter to fully concentrate on every repetition.

If you seek out the assistance of a professional trainer though, be meticulous. I would be remiss if I didn't clarify that the title "Certified Personal Trainer" means absolutely nothing in and of itself. There are *no* governing bodies, industry-wide standards, or state regulations for "Certified Personal Training Programs"—many certification programs do not even require a high school diploma. With more than 300 personal training certifications available, most on the Internet with official-sounding names, you'd be hard-pressed to find a well trained trainer. Don't trust your body to an unqualified trainer.

First and foremost, what does the person's physique look like? Although the trainer's physical appearance is not an indication of knowledge, trainers that stay in shape are fully vested into their profession. After all, you wouldn't take financial advice from a person on welfare, so why would you take fitness advice from someone that is out of shape? Next, what's their educational background? Not only in the field of fitness, but overall. Academic achievement can be a critical signal in the person's intellectual skills and attitude towards continued learning. I would recommend staying clear of any trainer with less than a four year college degree. One final note, does the person seem genuinely interested in you? A good trainer will be concerned about your medical history, taking into account any past injuries, and your personal fitness goals, not theirs. If you would like assistance in this area or information on workshops that I conduct for beginners, please visit my web site—**www.chazzweaver.com**.

The following exercises are not illustrated with paid twenty-year-old models, freshly made up, posing perfectly as the lights glisten off shiny chrome weights, demonstrating exercises that no beginner should execute. However, if you accurately follow the directions for each exercise, you will insure a firm foundation that will lead to real results. Each movement will be discussed from the vantage point of utilizing weight machines. A good gym or fitness center will have numerous weight machines set up to work each muscle in your body. Weight machines direct your body through the movement, eliminating the added task of having to balance free weights. Machines are great for beginners because they are less intimidating. You select a weight that is suitable for you and just follow the machine's range of motion to work the appropriate muscle. Since beginners are not yet skilled on proper form, these machines will help prevent injuries as they control the movements—all that is needed from the individual is to perform the movement with maximum intensity.

Chest Muscles

Chest Press—Lie or sit, depending on the machine, with your back flush against the bench and your upper chest under the lever bar. Grasp the bar with a wide overhand grip. Press the bar until your arms are extended then lower weight to your upper chest. Repeat the movement.

Back Muscles

Pull Downs—Sit with your thighs under the support pads. Grasp the overhead bar with a shoulder wide grip. Pull the bar down to your upper chest. Return until your arms and shoulders are fully extended. Repeat the movement.

Shoulder Muscles

Shoulder Press—Sit on the seat and grasp the bar with an overhand grip. Press the bar until your arms are extended overhead. Lower and repeat.

Arm Muscles

Seated Bicep Curls—Sit on the seat and grasp handles with an underhand grip. Position your elbows to sides so they are in line with bar's swivel. Raise the handles until your elbows are fully flexed with the back of your upper arms remaining on the pad. Lower handles until your arms are fully extended. Repeat. The biceps may be exercised alternating or simultaneous. If the machine does not provide support for the back of your arms, keep your elbows from traveling back, particularly during initial flexing.

Seated Triceps Extension—Sit on the seat. Grasp handles and place the backs of your upper arms on padding so that your elbows are in line with the lever's swivel. Push the lever down until your arms are fully extended. Return and repeat.

Leg Muscles

Leg Extensions—Sit on the machine with your back against the padded back support. Place the front of your lower legs under the padded lever. Position your knees at same axis as lever swivel. Grasp handles for support. Move the lever forward by straightening legs until legs are straight. Return lever to original position by bending knees. Repeat the movement. Stabilizers are used during heavy resistances to prevent the body from rising off of the seat.

Lying Leg Curls—Lie flat on the bench, face down, with knees just beyond the edge of the bench and lower legs under lever pads. Grasp handles. Raise lever pads to the back of your thighs by flexing knees. Lower lever pads until knees are straight. Repeat the movement. Keep your torso on the bench to reduce hyperextension of the lower back. Most machines are angled at the user's hip to position the hamstring in a more favorable mechanical position.

Standing Calf Raise—Place shoulders under the padded lever. Position toes and balls of your feet on the calf block with arches and heels extending off. Grasp handles or sides of padded lever. Stand erect by extending hips and knees. Raise heels by extending ankles as high as possible. Lower heels by bending ankles until calves are stretched. Repeat the movement.

The End of the Book, the Beginning of the Journey

At this point, you and I have traveled a long way together. If you have already begun to incorporate some of the changes and strategies that I have suggested into your life, congratulations. If you are still preparing for the major life change that implementing a healthier lifestyle will likely represent, I support your decision, because this is the kind of commitment that should not be entered into lightly. In order to ensure that you will succeed in your fitness and weight loss goals, it is important to come up with a viable plan and a strategy, along with contingency plans, that you will be able to stick to in the long-term.

We've covered a lot of ground together in this book. The concepts will form the foundation for the health and fitness plan which you will create. As I have said before, I feel strongly that *you* must be the person who devises your personal plan for weight loss success—I've just provided you with the knowledge and tools that will allow you to make an effective plan based on my proven template.

The majority of the fad diet books on the market today set out strict guidelines, even going as far as creating menus for each meal. I know, and you know as well, that real life rarely permits that level of inflexibility. Instead, you have to be able to develop and stick to a plan that is adaptable enough to see you through the unexpected twists and turns that make up everyday life.

That is why the fitness strategy that I have demonstrated over the course of this book is highly flexible and adaptable to the everyday challenges of life. So flexible, in fact, that you can even eat fast-food, from McDonald's or from another comparable establishment, and still lose weight, as I demonstrated as part of this project. This will work for you, too, as long as you have done a little research about the nutritional values of the food offerings at any establishment you choose and you make strong food choices when you are presented with that kind of situation.

The tools that we've gone over so far have included basic nutrition through caloric value, aerobic and anaerobic exercise, and motivation. There's one more key ingredient that we haven't really talked about yet, but I'd like to think I've been modeling the way it can be applied to the weight loss process throughout the course of this book. That ingredient is rational thinking, and that's the reason why it took an economist to write this book.

As I have mentioned, my formal training is in the field of economics, a discipline in which I have earned a master's degree. Yet, my body has been the laboratory I've used to develop successful ideas and strategies for overall fitness. I have since worked with many other individuals who have applied these ideas with great accomplishment.

At first glance, the field of economics might seem to have little to do with weight loss. In fact, if you're anything like most people, you probably associate the field of economics with the issues of finance, stock markets, gross national products, and deficits. But, in reality, these topics just constitute one small aspect of economics. Actually, the tools that economists are trained to use can lend a new perspective to many different problems, including the problem of obesity and the challenge of weight loss.

Although many economists spend most of their time thinking about financial issues, all that economics really boils down to is the use of a special set of analytical tools to identify problems, point out differences, similarities, and patterns in order to devise solutions to many different kinds of situations and dilemmas. While this aspect of economics is still relatively unknown to the general public, it's become more prominent in recent years.

Recently, in fact, one of the most promising up-and-coming American economists, Steven Levitt, released a *New York Times* best selling book called *Freakonomics* that highlighted the usefulness of economics as a problem-solving tool. Although economics is not the kind of subject matter that you usually associate with massive popularity amidst mainstream American readers, Levitt's book captured a wide-ranging audience.

In *Freakonomics*, Levitt and his co-author, Stephen Dubner, describe the many ways that the tools of economics can be applied to everyday problems to gain a clearer understanding of the issue and devise new solutions. The challenges that Levitt has tackled in his career have ranged from identifying teachers who were helping their students cheat on standardized tests, ascertaining the salary earned by street gang members, to analyzing the unusual marketing techniques and propaganda methods used by hate groups like the Ku Klux Klan.

The prospect of using the tools of economics to talk about weight loss, fitness, and the obesity problem facing the United States today doesn't seem quite as unusual now, does it? Throughout most of this book, I've talked to you as a fellow traveler on the journey towards increased health, fitness, and quality of life. Now, for a few moments before we part ways, I'd like to talk to you as an economist.

Wait, don't run away! I'm not going to bore you to tears talking about historical stock market performance and the import/export trade deficit! Like I said before, all that the term "economics" refers to is looking at problems from a certain analytical perspective. Although a lot of specialists in economics happen to focus on issues of finance, you can use these same basic tools and strategies to take a look at any problem that you may be facing.

Remember, I am a big believer in looking at problems from a simple analytical perspective, such as the maxim that holds that if you consume fewer calories than you expend, you will lose weight. The same holds true for using the laws of economics to look at the problem of obesity, both on a personal and a societal level.

The costs of obesity are staggering. Every year, the negative outcomes associated with our nation's growing weight problem increases and accumulates. It is estimated that obesity contributes directly and indirectly to nearly a half a million deaths annually. In financial terms, nearly $100 billion annually is spent on health care costs that are linked directly to obesity. Add this to the nearly $50 billion that Americans invest in new forms of diet and health related products and paraphernalia, and you can see that this problem is costing the country a staggering amount of money.

But what about the non-financial costs that are associated with obesity in the United States and elsewhere in the world? I would argue that despite the billions of dollars that we spend on the obesity problem, it pales in comparison to the huge emotional, social, behavioral, and even cultural toll that obesity has taken upon us as a people.

Although obesity is not solely to blame for phenomena like the lack of physical activity, declines in the time families spend together, and spiraling rates of childhood illness, it plays a role in all of these problems, as well as contributing to many other undesirable aspects of twenty-first century life. More people, particularly Americans, are obese today than at any other time in history, and the lack of freedom, mobility, and self-confidence that are all too often the sad byproducts of obesity have left a permanent mark on each culture.

As an economist, it is not difficult to understand how obesity has become a problem of unprecedented scope in recent years. As the processes of food production, manufacturing, and distribution have been refined in recent years, food prices have fallen. Although it may seem as if your grocery bill is higher than ever before, our grocery dollar goes further in terms of the amount of calories it will buy than it did in the past. As a result, we can eat more calories for less money.

However, while economics can readily explain why obesity has become a problem at the level of society, the issue becomes more complex at the level of the individual. For most people, being obese or overweight is an undesirable state of affairs. Most people who are currently obese or overweight would tell you, if asked, that they would rather be fit, healthy, and slim.

And yet, few take the actions that are necessary to achieve this goal. Instead, many of us choose to continue with our long-held unhealthy habits, eating poorly and exercising rarely, if at all, pouring money into fad diets that are never successful in the long-term.

From an economic standpoint, from a perspective of rational thinking, this approach simply does not make sense. If you desire an outcome, such as increased health, you should take the course of action that is most likely to result in your achieving that outcome, while avoiding actions that are likely to impede or undermine your efforts. *You must make the choice to make the change and stick with it.*

You can try to use all of the emotional or psychological justifications that you can come up with, but it simply does not make sense to fail to act in a manner that is consistent with the outcome that you desire. I know that you understand that, both in your mind and in your heart, even if it hurts to hear it. Choosing to do nothing is also a choice, just as sure as choosing to change your life is.

I challenge you to start today. Make the choice to begin making strides toward your goal. *Every little baby step counts.* Don't think about the whole, overwhelming process at once. Just commit to one day of exercise, one day of strong food choices, and one day of healthy living; and then, to one more day; and then to another. Be flexible and adaptable, and remember that this plan will see you through the unexpected twists and turns of everyday life. Just don't give up, even if you have a bad day. Even if you have a bad week, don't give up. Before you know it, you will be well on your way to a new you and a new life.

Endnotes

1 McGuire et al A 30-year follow-up of the Dallas bed rest and training study: Effect of age on the cardiovascular response to exercise. Circulation 2001; 104:1350-7.

2 McGuire et al A 30-year follow-up of the Dallas bed rest and training study: Effect of age on the cardiovascular response to exercise. Circulation 2001; 104:1350-7.

3 Blix, G.G. & Blix, A.G. (1998). The role of exercise in weight loss. Behavioral Medicine, 21(1), 31-39.

4 Hansen, K., Shriver, T. & Schoeller, D. (2005). The effects of exercise on the storage and oxidation of dietary fat. Sports Medicine, 35(5), 363-373.

5 Blix, G.G. & Blix, A.G. (1998). The role of exercise in weight loss. Behavioral Medicine, 21(1), 31-39.

6 Blix, G.G. & Blix, A.G. (1998). The role of exercise in weight loss. Behavioral Medicine, 21(1), 31-39.

7 Blix, G.G. & Blix, A.G. (1998). The role of exercise in weight loss. Behavioral Medicine, 21(1), 31-39.

8 Hansen, K., Shriver, T. & Schoeller, D. (2005). The effects of exercise on the storage and oxidation of dietary fat. Sports Medicine, 35(5), 363-373.

9 Blix, G.G. & Blix, A.G. (1998). The role of exercise in weight loss. Behavioral Medicine, 21(1), 31-39.

10 Blix, G.G. & Blix, A.G. (1998). The role of exercise in weight loss. Behavioral Medicine, 21(1), 31-39.

11 Blix, G.G. & Blix, A.G. (1998). The role of exercise in weight loss. Behavioral Medicine, 21(1), 31-39.

12 Nied, R.J. (2002). Promoting and prescribing exercise for the elderly. American Family Physician, 65(3), 419-426.

13 Blix, G.G. & Blix, A.G. (1998). The role of exercise in weight loss. Behavioral Medicine, 21(1), 31-39.

14 Ritchie, C.S., Stetson, B.A., Bass, P.F. & Adams, K.J. (2002). Talking to patients about aerobic exercise for disease prevention. Nutrition in Clinical Care, 5(3), 103-104.

15 Elley, C.R. & Arroll, B. (2002). Aerobic exercise reduces systolic and diastolic blood pressure in adults. ACP Journal, 137(3), 109.

16 Ritchie, C.S., Stetson, B.A., Bass, P.F. & Adams, K.J. (2002). Talking to patients about aerobic exercise for disease prevention. Nutrition in Clinical Care, 5(3), 103-104.

17 Blix, G.G. & Blix, A.G. (1998). The role of exercise in weight loss. Behavioral Medicine, 21(1), 31-39.

18 Nied, R.J. (2002). Promoting and prescribing exercise for the elderly. American Family Physician, 65(3), 419-426.

19 Blix, G.G. & Blix, A.G. (1998). The role of exercise in weight loss. Behavioral Medicine, 21(1), 31-39.

20 Hansen, K., Shriver, T. & Schoeller, D. (2005). The effects of exercise on the storage and oxidation of dietary fat. Sports Medicine, 35(5), 363-373.

21 Hansen, K., Shriver, T. & Schoeller, D. (2005). The effects of exercise on the storage and oxidation of dietary fat. Sports Medicine, 35(5), 363-373.

22 Blix, G.G. & Blix, A.G. (1998). The role of exercise in weight loss. Behavioral Medicine, 21(1), 31-39.

23 Hansen, K., Shriver, T. & Schoeller, D. (2005). The effects of exercise on the storage and oxidation of dietary fat. Sports Medicine, 35(5), 363-373.

24 Hansen, K., Shriver, T. & Schoeller, D. (2005). The effects of exercise on the storage and oxidation of dietary fat. Sports Medicine, 35(5), 363-373.

25 Hansen, K., Shriver, T. & Schoeller, D. (2005). The effects of exercise on the storage and oxidation of dietary fat. Sports Medicine, 35(5), 363-373.

26 Blix, G.G. & Blix, A.G. (1998). The role of exercise in weight loss. Behavioral Medicine, 21(1), 31-39.

27 Kraemer, W.J. & Knuttgen, H.G. (2003). Strength training basics. Physician & Sports Medicine, 31(8), 39-45.

28 Kraemer, W.J. & Knuttgen, H.G. (2003). Strength training basics. Physician & Sports Medicine, 31(8), 39-45.

29 Kraemer, W.J. & Knuttgen, H.G. (2003). Strength training basics. Physician & Sports Medicine, 31(8), 39-45.

30 Kraemer, W.J. & Knuttgen, H.G. (2003). Strength training basics. Physician & Sports Medicine, 31(8), 39-45.

31 Kraemer, W.J. & Knuttgen, H.G. (2003). Strength training basics. Physician & Sports Medicine, 31(8), 39-45.

32 Hoff, J. & Helgerud, J. (2004). Endurance and strength training for soccer players: Physiological considerations. Sports Medicine, 34(3), 165-180.

33 Hoff, J. & Helgerud, J. (2004). Endurance and strength training for soccer players: Physiological considerations. Sports Medicine, 34(3), 165-180.

34 Hoff, J. & Helgerud, J. (2004). Endurance and strength training for soccer players: Physiological considerations. Sports Medicine, 34(3), 165-180.

35 Nied, R.J. (2002). Promoting and prescribing exercise for the elderly. American Family Physician, 65(3), 419-426.

36 Hoff, J. & Helgerud, J. (2004). Endurance and strength training for soccer players: Physiological considerations. Sports Medicine, 34(3), 165-180.

37 Nied, R.J. (2002). Promoting and prescribing exercise for the elderly. American Family Physician, 65(3), 419-426.

38 Kruger, J., Brown, D.R., Galuska, D.A. & Buchner, D. (2004). Strength training among adults aged ≥65 years--United States, 2001. Morbidity & Mortality Weekly Report, 53(2), 25-28.

39 Nied, R.J. (2002). Promoting and prescribing exercise for the elderly. American Family Physician, 65(3), 419-426; Rosario, E.J., Villani, R.G., Harris, J. & Klein, R. (2003). Comparison of strength-training adaptations in early and older menopausal women. Journal of Aging & Physical Activity, 11(2), 143-155.

40 Nied, R.J. (2002). Promoting and prescribing exercise for the elderly. American Family Physician, 65(3), 419-426.

41 Bartlett, S.J. (2003). Motivating patients toward weight loss. Physician & Sports Medicine, 31(11), 29-36.

42 White, F. (2004). Identifying and treating exercise resistance from a depth perspective. Health at Every Size, 18(4), 58-60.

43 White, F. (2004). Identifying and treating exercise resistance from a depth perspective. Health at Every Size, 18(4), 58-60.

44 Gallucci, N.T. (1995). The effects of goals on the maintenance of exercise programs. Journal of Sport Behavior, 18(2), 109-122.

45 Lustyk, M.B., Widman, L., Paschane, A.A.E. & Olson, K.C. (2004). Physical activity and quality of life: Assessing the influence of activity frequency, intensity, volume, and motives. Behavioral Medicine, 30(3), 124-131.

46 Gavin, J. (2004). Pairing personality with activity. Physician & Sports Medicine, 32(12), 17-24.

47 Lustyk, M.B., Widman, L., Paschane, A.A.E. & Olson, K.C. (2004). Physical activity and quality of life: Assessing the influence of activity frequency, intensity, volume, and motives. Behavioral Medicine, 30(3), 124-131.

48 Gavin, J. (2004). Pairing personality with activity. Physician & Sports Medicine, 32(12), 17-24.

49 Bartlett, S.J. (2003). Motivating patients toward weight loss. Physician & Sports Medicine, 31(11), 29-36.

50 Bartlett, S.J. (2003). Motivating patients toward weight loss. Physician & Sports Medicine, 31(11), 29-36.

51 Kilpatrick, M., Hebert, E. & Bartholomew, J. (2005). College studentsí motivation for physical activity: Differentiating menís and womenís motives for sport participation and exercise. Journal of American College Health, 54(2), 87-94.

52 Bartlett, S.J. (2003). Motivating patients toward weight loss. Physician & Sports Medicine, 31(11), 29-36.

53 Bartlett, S.J. (2003). Motivating patients toward weight loss. Physician & Sports Medicine, 31(11), 29-36.

54 Gallucci, N.T. (1995). The effects of goals on the maintenance of exercise programs. Journal of Sport Behavior, 18(2), 109-122.

55 Young, T.D. (2005). Factors determining exercise adherence. American Fitness, 23(1), 46-50.

56 Volek, J.S., Van Heest, J.L. & Forsythe, C.E. (2005). Diet and exercise for weight loss: A review of current issues. Sports Medicine, 35(1), 1-9.

57 Young, T.D. (2005). Factors determining exercise adherence. American Fitness, 23(1), 46-50.

58 Paxton, S.J. & Sculthorpe, A. (1999). Weight and health locus of control beliefs in an Australian community sample. Psychology & Health, 14(3), 417-431.

59 Young, T.D. (2005). Factors determining exercise adherence. American Fitness, 23(1), 46-50.

60 Gallucci, N.T. (1995). The effects of goals on the maintenance of exercise programs. Journal of Sport Behavior, 18(2), 109-122.

61 Paxton, S.J. & Sculthorpe, A. (1999). Weight and health locus of control beliefs in an Australian community sample. Psychology & Health, 14(3), 417-431.

62 Kilpatrick, M., Hebert, E. & Bartholomew, J. (2005). College studentsí motivation for physical activity: Differentiating menís and womenís motives for sport participation and exercise. Journal of American College Health, 54(2), 87-94.

63 Dacey, M.L. (2005). A client-centered counseling approach for motivating older adults toward physical activity. Topics in Geriatric Rehabilitation, 21(3), 194-205.

64 Kilpatrick, M., Hebert, E. & Bartholomew, J. (2005). College studentsí motivation for physical activity: Differentiating menís and womenís motives for sport participation and exercise. Journal of American College Health, 54(2), 87-94.

65 Young, T.D. (2005). Factors determining exercise adherence. American Fitness, 23(1), 46-50.

FOR MORE INFORMATION

www.chazzweaver.com
www.truthinfitness.org

DAILY FITNESS JOURNAL

TRAINING LOG / FOOD LOG

TRAINING LOG

Date____________________

Aerobic Exercise	Total Time
Example - Stationary Bike - at level 4	*20 min.*

Strength Training (Note: Reps/Weight = 1 set)	**Set #1** Reps/Weight	**Set #2** Reps/Weight	**Set #3** Reps/Weight	**Set #4** Reps/Weight
Example – Chest Press	*15reps/25lbs*	*15/25*	*12/25*	*12/25*

Daily Comments:

FOOD LOG

Date

Time	Food/Beverage	Calories
Example		
7:00am	*6 egg whites with 2 yokes*	*242*
Meal #1, Omelette	*4 oz Chicken Breast*	*120*
	Grape Tomatoes & Mushrooms	*40*
	Black Coffee	*0*

Total Calories – 402

Total Daily Calories

TRAINING LOG

Date

Aerobic Exercise

Total Time

Strength Training (Note: Reps/Weight = 1 set)	**Set #1** Reps/Weight	**Set #2** Reps/Weight	**Set #3** Reps/Weight	**Set #4** Reps/Weight

Daily Comments:

FOOD LOG

Date

Time	Food/Beverage	Calories

Total Daily Calories

TRAINING LOG

Date

Aerobic Exercise

Total Time

Strength Training (Note: Reps/Weight = 1 set)	**Set #1 Reps/Weight**	**Set #2 Reps/Weight**	**Set #3 Reps/Weight**	**Set #4 Reps/Weight**

Daily Comments:

FOOD LOG

Date

Time	Food/Beverage	Calories

Total Daily Calories

TRAINING LOG

Date

Aerobic Exercise | Total Time

Strength Training (Note: Reps/Weight = 1 set) | **Set #1** Reps/Weight | **Set #2** Reps/Weight | **Set #3** Reps/Weight | **Set #4** Reps/Weight

Daily Comments:

FOOD LOG

Date

Time	Food/Beverage	Calories

Total Daily Calories

TRAINING LOG

Date

Aerobic Exercise

Total Time

Strength Training (Note: Reps/Weight = 1 set)	**Set #1** Reps/Weight	**Set #2** Reps/Weight	**Set #3** Reps/Weight	**Set #4** Reps/Weight

Daily Comments:

FOOD LOG

Date

Time	Food/Beverage	Calories

Total Daily Calories

TRAINING LOG

Date

Aerobic Exercise | Total Time

Strength Training (Note: Reps/Weight = 1 set)	**Set #1** Reps/Weight	**Set #2** Reps/Weight	**Set #3** Reps/Weight	**Set #4** Reps/Weight

Daily Comments:

FOOD LOG

Date

Time	Food/Beverage	Calories

Total Daily Calories

TRAINING LOG

Date

Aerobic Exercise | Total Time

Strength Training (Note: Reps/Weight = 1 set)	**Set #1** Reps/Weight	**Set #2** Reps/Weight	**Set #3** Reps/Weight	**Set #4** Reps/Weight

Daily Comments:

FOOD LOG

Date

Time	Food/Beverage	Calories

Total Daily Calories

TRAINING LOG

Date

Aerobic Exercise

Total Time

Strength Training (Note: Reps/Weight = 1 set)	**Set #1** Reps/Weight	**Set #2** Reps/Weight	**Set #3** Reps/Weight	**Set #4** Reps/Weight

Daily Comments:

FOOD LOG

Date

Time	Food/Beverage	Calories

Total Daily Calories

TRAINING LOG

Date

Aerobic Exercise

Total Time

Strength Training (Note: Reps/Weight = 1 set)	**Set #1** Reps/Weight	**Set #2** Reps/Weight	**Set #3** Reps/Weight	**Set #4** Reps/Weight

Daily Comments:

FOOD LOG

Date

Time	Food/Beverage	Calories

Total Daily Calories

TRAINING LOG

Date

Aerobic Exercise

Total Time

Strength Training **(Note: Reps/Weight = 1 set)**	**Set #1** **Reps/Weight**	**Set #2** **Reps/Weight**	**Set #3** **Reps/Weight**	**Set #4** **Reps/Weight**

Daily Comments:

FOOD LOG

Date

Time	Food/Beverage	Calories

Total Daily Calories

TRAINING LOG

Date

Aerobic Exercise

Total Time

Strength Training (Note: Reps/Weight = 1 set)	**Set #1** Reps/Weight	**Set #2** Reps/Weight	**Set #3** Reps/Weight	**Set #4** Reps/Weight

Daily Comments:

FOOD LOG

Date____________________

Time	Food/Beverage	Calories

Total Daily Calories____________________

TRAINING LOG

Date

Aerobic Exercise

Total Time

Strength Training (Note: Reps/Weight = 1 set)	**Set #1** Reps/Weight	**Set #2** Reps/Weight	**Set #3** Reps/Weight	**Set #4** Reps/Weight

Daily Comments:

FOOD LOG

Date

Time	Food/Beverage	Calories

Total Daily Calories

TRAINING LOG

Date

Aerobic Exercise

Total Time

Strength Training (Note: Reps/Weight = 1 set)	**Set #1** Reps/Weight	**Set #2** Reps/Weight	**Set #3** Reps/Weight	**Set #4** Reps/Weight

Daily Comments:

FOOD LOG

Date

Time	Food/Beverage	Calories

Total Daily Calories

TRAINING LOG

Date ______________________

Aerobic Exercise | Total Time

Strength Training (Note: Reps/Weight = 1 set)	Set #1 Reps/Weight	Set #2 Reps/Weight	Set #3 Reps/Weight	Set #4 Reps/Weight

Daily Comments:

FOOD LOG

Date

Time	Food/Beverage	Calories

Total Daily Calories

TRAINING LOG

Date

Aerobic Exercise

Total Time

Strength Training (Note: Reps/Weight = 1 set)	**Set #1** Reps/Weight	**Set #2** Reps/Weight	**Set #3** Reps/Weight	**Set #4** Reps/Weight

Daily Comments:

FOOD LOG

Date

Time	Food/Beverage	Calories

Total Daily Calories

TRAINING LOG

Date

Aerobic Exercise | Total Time

Strength Training (Note: Reps/Weight = 1 set)	**Set #1** Reps/Weight	**Set #2** Reps/Weight	**Set #3** Reps/Weight	**Set #4** Reps/Weight

Daily Comments:

FOOD LOG

Date

Time	Food/Beverage	Calories

Total Daily Calories

TRAINING LOG

Date

Aerobic Exercise

Total Time

Strength Training (Note: Reps/Weight = 1 set)	**Set #1 Reps/Weight**	**Set #2 Reps/Weight**	**Set #3 Reps/Weight**	**Set #4 Reps/Weight**

Daily Comments:

FOOD LOG

Date

Time	Food/Beverage	Calories

Total Daily Calories

TRAINING LOG

Date

Aerobic Exercise | Total Time

Strength Training (Note: Reps/Weight = 1 set)	**Set #1** Reps/Weight	**Set #2** Reps/Weight	**Set #3** Reps/Weight	**Set #4** Reps/Weight

Daily Comments:

FOOD LOG

Date

Time	Food/Beverage	Calories

Total Daily Calories

TRAINING LOG

Date

Aerobic Exercise | Total Time

Strength Training (Note: Reps/Weight = 1 set)	**Set #1** Reps/Weight	**Set #2** Reps/Weight	**Set #3** Reps/Weight	**Set #4** Reps/Weight

Daily Comments:

FOOD LOG

Date

Time	Food/Beverage	Calories

Total Daily Calories

TRAINING LOG

Date

Aerobic Exercise

Total Time

Strength Training (Note: Reps/Weight = 1 set)	**Set #1** Reps/Weight	**Set #2** Reps/Weight	**Set #3** Reps/Weight	**Set #4** Reps/Weight

Daily Comments:

FOOD LOG

Date

Time	Food/Beverage	Calories

Total Daily Calories

TRAINING LOG

Date

Aerobic Exercise

Total Time

Strength Training **(Note: Reps/Weight = 1 set)**	**Set #1** **Reps/Weight**	**Set #2** **Reps/Weight**	**Set #3** **Reps/Weight**	**Set #4** **Reps/Weight**

Daily Comments:

FOOD LOG

Date____________________

Time	Food/Beverage	Calories

Total Daily Calories____________________

TATE PUBLISHING & *Enterprises*

Tate Publishing is committed to excellence in the publishing industry. Our staff of highly trained professionals, including editors, graphic designers, and marketing personnel, work together to produce the very finest books available. The company reflects the philosophy established by the founders, based on Psalms 68:11,

"THE LORD GAVE THE WORD AND GREAT WAS THE COMPANY OF THOSE WHO PUBLISHED IT."

If you would like further information, please call
1.888.361.9473
or visit our website
www.tatepublishing.com

TATE PUBLISHING & *Enterprises*, LLC
127 E. Trade Center Terrace
Mustang, Oklahoma 73064 USA